LSD
SPIRITUALITY
AND THE
CREATIVE
PROCESS

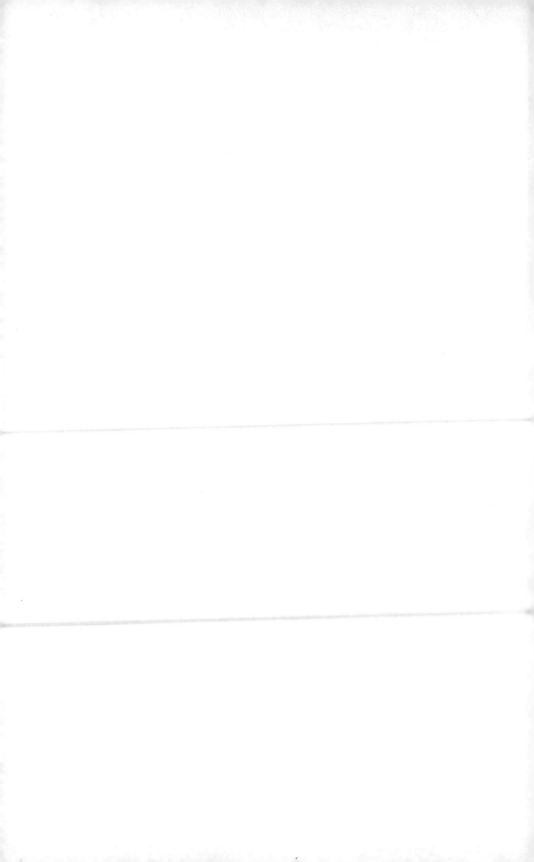

LSD
SPIRITUALITY
AND THE
CREATIVE
PROCESS

**Marlene Dobkin de Rios, Ph.D.
and Oscar Janiger, M.D.**

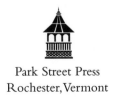

Park Street Press
Rochester, Vermont

Park Street Press
One Park Street
Rochester, Vermont 05767
www.InnerTraditions.com

Park Street Press is a division of Inner Traditions International

Library of Congress Cataloging-in-Publication Data
Dobkin de Rios, Marlene.
  LSD, spirituality, and the creative process / Marlene Dobkin de Rios
and Oscar Janiger.
     p. ; cm.
Includes bibliographical references and index.
  ISBN 0-89281-973-1
  1. LSD (Drug)--Longitudinal studies. 2. Creative ability. 3.
Creation (Literary, artistic, etc.) 4. Spiritual life.
  [DNLM: 1. Lysergic Acid Diethylamide--pharmacology. 2. Creativeness.
3. Hallucinogens--pharmacology. 4. Longitudinal Studies. QV 77.7
D633L 2003] I. Janiger, Oscar. II. Title.
  BF209.L9 D57 2003
  154.4--dc21

2003004254

Printed and bound in the United States by Lake Book Manufacturing, Inc.

10 9 8 7 6 5 4 3 2 1

Text design and layout by Priscilla Baker
This book was typeset in Bembo, with Schneidler and Avenir as display typefaces

This book is dedicated to the memory of Dr. Oscar Janiger,
dear friend and adviser.

CONTENTS

ACKNOWLEDGMENTS

MANY THANKS for the gracious assistance of Professor Carl Hertel, whose clarity of vision has been of enormous help in understanding the creative process. Thanks are also due to David Smith, M.D., founder and director of the Haight Ashbury Free Clinic, and Richard Seymour, for their encouragement in providing a forum for unfettered discussion. I would like to acknowledge the good offices and help of the Multidisciplinary Association for Psychedelic Studies (MAPS) for their hard work and determination in completing the follow-up study of Janiger's original research. And to the many artists and participants in this study, a special thanks for your courage and valor in uncharted waters.

FOREWORD

I AM DELIGHTED to be associated with the publication of *LSD, Spirituality, and the Creative Process*. This book recounts Dr. Oscar Janiger's remarkable studies of the effects of LSD on humans, conducted during the 1950's and early 1960's, which have been lying unappreciated for too long. Even more important than the fact that these studies are finally coming to light, however, is the unique nature of their data. Janiger investigated the effects of LSD using a model that was markedly different from the prevailing one. As a result, what he sought and discovered stands out in stark contrast relative to other studies taking place at that time.

Most research with psychedelic drugs in humans occurred in hospital-based clinical research settings. Subjects were often mentally ill, received little information about LSD's expected effects, and underwent intrusive monitoring and testing. The very design of such experiment-based research was bound to influence one's response to the drug. Janiger's work provided a striking alternative to this model.

Using a comfortable home setting and common-sense preparation of volunteers, he gave nearly 1000 curious and psychologically ordinary volunteers this powerful hallucinogen. He provided a safe and relatively non-directive environment for allowing the drug's effects to unfold, and collected a vast number of volunteer self-reports. Overall, it is impressive how positive are the descriptions of volunteers' sessions, how rare is the occurrence of adverse effects, and how enduring is the memory of one's participation in the study.

Psychedelics, perhaps more so than any other family of psychoactive drugs, exert their effects through a confluence of *pharmacology, set,* and *setting*. This inextricable dependence upon set and setting is why we hear such widely divergent reports about what LSD does, even in the same person at the same dose, but on different days and in different circumstances. This is also why there are so many different names used to label LSD and related drugs; for example, *psychedelic* (mind-manifesting), *hallucinogenic* (producing hallucinations), *psychotomimetic* (mimicking psychosis), and *entheogenic* (manifesting the intrinsically divine).

Burdensome regulations enacted in the United States in 1970 resulted in a twenty-year interruption of human research with psychedelic drugs. Nevertheless, the prevalence of their use never significantly fell, and they are as popular as ever among adolescents and young adults in the West. In addition, "underground" therapists employ them as adjuncts to their work with clients, indigenous shamanic use is increasingly popular, and religious organizations using psychedelic plant sacraments challenge our notions of spirituality and drug use.

When Janiger began his work publicity, especially the frightening misleading type, was minimal regarding LSD's effects. However it is not accurate to say that Janiger's work was free of bias. Rather, it reflected his own biases and those of his colleagues—a more hopeful and forward-thinking perspective and approach toward these drugs that unfortunately received little exposure. Now Marlene Dobkin de Rios thoroughly sifts through, compiles, and classifies the results that emerged from Janiger's uniquely supportive and non-directive administration of LSD. She also weaves through them a valuable broad perspective obtained through decades of her anthropologic research into the use of psychedelic plants.

With the recent resumption of government-approved studies of psychedelic drugs in humans, our larger culture again faces the question of how to understand these drugs' effects. The "psychotomimetic" and "psychedelic" viewpoints remain as valid, and potentially contentious, as they did 50 years ago. Any serious discussion of how to approach the study of these fascinating but controversial drugs will only be benefited by including Janiger's work, which is now available to us.

Rick J. Strassman M.D., Clinical Associate Professor of Psychiatry,
University of New Mexico School of Medicine
Author of *DMT: The Spirit Molecule*
www.rickstrassman.com

INTRODUCTION

THE YEAR IS 1954. Los Angeles psychiatrist Oscar Janiger is permitted by the Swiss pharmaceutical corporation Sandoz to experiment with the relatively new substance called LSD-25. The curious come to imbibe, and by the end of an eight-year period that ends abruptly by government fiat in 1962, Dr. Janiger has given LSD-25 to more than 930 men and women, ranging in age from eighteen to eighty-one. Some are teachers and professionals, some are housewives, some are truckers, some construction workers, and some are unemployed. All take a measured dose of pure LSD, provided by Sandoz Corporation, and all are given the substance in a controlled and safe environment—a private home rented for the experiment by Dr. Janiger. All agree to allow their experiences to be recorded and to participate in follow-up requests for information on the LSD's long-term effects, if any, on their lives.

Janiger's general aim was to explore and study the effects of LSD on a large, highly differentiated group of people in a natural setting. Initially, Janiger sought simply to discover what LSD does to an average person. Is there, he wondered, such a thing as an intrinsic, characteristic LSD response? If so, what is it? In fact, the volunteers' experiences varied widely, although Janiger did identify some twenty-eight common responses that he considered core characteristics of the LSD experience.

Beyond his general curiosity in the LSD response, however, Janiger also brought to his work a defined interest in LSD's therapeutic use—although his study was not constructed to test its validity. As his research progressed Janiger also grew interested in LSD's influence on creativity, and he developed a parallel study to examine the influence of a psychedelic on the creative process in a controlled setting. In one of the few studies of its kind, sixty professional artists took LSD under Janiger's guidance during the early years of his research. And finally, although he never intended to study LSD's relationship to spiritual experience, Janiger found the connection to be inescapable.

This study was unique in the size and diversity of its sample. While some researchers of this period worked with a small number of subjects in hospital settings and found pure pathology emerging from their subjects' reports, Janiger's volunteers represented a generous cross-section of American society, including housewives, cooks, cashiers, professionals, constructions workers, artists, and writers. Janiger was amazed at his participants' eloquent and insightful responses to the substance. It was as if he had assembled in one place a large number of unusually interesting men and women with profound philosophical leanings—instead of mostly ordinary folks. Certainly no other study was sustained as long or yielded as much and as wide-ranging information as this experiment.

Janiger's research took place at a moment in history that can truly never be repeated, a time that was uncontaminated by either expectation or hype, when there was little knowledge or understanding of the effects of this powerful substance and its influence in deconditioning the individual from his or her strongly-held beliefs, values, and ways of thinking and feeling. Moreover, while this was by no means the only study where artists were given LSD (see ten Berge 2002 for discussions of several early experiments with artists and hallucinogens) the large number of artists, writers, and musicians who participated in Janiger's study was noteworthy. The artwork and poetry they produced were collected, and samples of this work are displayed in appendices II and IV.

Unique as the study was, it nevertheless came to an abrupt halt in 1962, when an FDA representative came to see Janiger and required him to turn over all the stock of LSD. Janiger, along with other LSD researchers, protested that no laws had been broken and that the FDA demand was illegal. Nonetheless, Janiger and his counterparts all complied with the order, and he canceled all outstanding appointments.

As upset as Janiger and many of his colleagues were at what they felt was an unjustified indictment and interruption of important work, the tide of public perception had turned against them. By 1962 the media uproar about LSD had begun in response to uncontrolled experimentation by young people and sensationalized reports of negative effects. Timothy Leary's self-proclaimed and surprisingly seductive mission to use LSD to "turn on and tune out" the world further discredited LSD's legitimate role in clinical research. Sandoz Corporation released all of their LSD materials, stopped production, and washed their hands of the LSD business. Responding to the restriction on medical use of LSD, the head of the company was reputed to have said: "Can you believe such a thing?" Had clinical researchers been able to prove the medical use of LSD they would have protected the substance, as occurred with Ketamine, which is an anesthetic as well as a psychedelic in its effects. Although Ketamine has an abuse potential, it is very much in evidence as an anesthesia in burn units all around the world. But LSD's possible medical applications had yet to be determined, so its fate was sealed.

In 1969 Oscar Janiger began a long friendship with the author, a medical anthropologist, who studied the use of LSD-like plants in tribal and industrializing third-world societies, particularly in the South American Amazon. Janiger was interested in the way that psychedelic experience patterned within American society compared with tribal and third-world cultures' use of LSD-like substances and how other cultures minimized the so-called bad trip. In 1979 he traveled to the Peruvian Amazon city of Pucallpa to spend time with the author as she studied don Hildebrando Rios, a healer who used the hallucinogen ayahuasca to treat his clients' psychological illnesses. For her part, the author was fascinated to explore with Janiger what the similarities and differences in their research conclusions had to say about the impact of culture on people's psychedelic experiences. This book was inspired by interviews that the author conducted with Dr. Janiger over a five-month period between March 2001 and early August 2001, the time of his death. Many of the observations about the LSD constants and about the creative process that appear in this book have been directly incorporated from his notes.

In the author's view, the results of Janiger's study clearly suggest LSD's potential to heighten creative response, to instigate or deepen spiritual connection or awareness, and to aid in therapeutic processes. Today, there is a mild renaissance in the use of LSD-like substances in psychotherapy and research, after a forty-year period during which there has been virtually no research involving human subjects and LSD. A few scientists are poised to begin examining LSD's medical potential for treating refractory mental illnesses, drug and alcohol addiction, and anxiety associated with terminal illness. In fact, in October 2002 the FDA approved a proposal by Dr. Charles Grob, a psychiatrist, to conduct a pilot investigation to examine the safety and efficacy of psilocybin, a related hallucinogen, in the treatment of anxiety, depression, and pain associated with end-stage cancer.

In this climate of new possibilities, it is hoped that this chronicle of Janiger's early LSD research will generate greater interest and support for such worthwhile projects. With a follow-up study of the original volunteers recently conducted, and in homage to Dr. Janiger, the time appears right for a detailed reconsideration and evaluation of his pioneering work.

A NOTE REGARDING STUDY PARTICIPANTS' IDENTITIES

Care has been taken to avoid divulging the identities of the study participants. The initials of the volunteers' identities were chosen from a table of random numbers so as to prevent reconstructing the original initials. Genders were retained but significant others' names were changed to protect the identity of the volunteer. Files were and have been kept under lock and key with limited access, first in the custody of Dr. Janiger and subsequently with heirs and with me. The names of notables who participated in the study were not included in the book to protect their privacy.

1

A BRIEF HISTORY OF LSD RESEARCH

MANY PEOPLE KNOW THE STORY about the chemist Albert Hofmann, who in 1943 worked in the Swiss Sandoz Laboratories on certain derivatives of lysergic acid (from ergot). He became strangely ill and wrote in his laboratory journal: "I was seized by a peculiar sensation of vertigo and restlessness. Objects, as well as the shape of my associates in the laboratory, appeared to undergo optical changes. I was unable to concentrate on my work. In a dream-like state, I left for home. . . . [I] fell into a peculiar state of drunkenness characterized by an exaggerated imagination. With my eyes closed, fantastic pictures of extraordinary plasticity and intensive color seemed to surge towards me. After two hours, this state gradually subsided" (Hofmann 1980).

Hofmann was describing the now commonly known sensations that characterize LSD experiences. (Later in this chapter, we will see a more detailed description of the effects of LSD.) LSD had first been synthesized from ergot in 1938 by Dr. W. A. Stoll, then the director of the Sandoz Laboratories. Hofmann accidentally discovered the hallucinogenic effects of the substance while he was trying to find a way to prevent nausea in people who took ergot to control migraine pain.

EARLY RESEARCH

Psychiatrists quickly became interested in the potential therapeutic use of this potent substance. In the period between 1943 and 1947, Stoll's son, a psychiatrist, gave LSD to advanced schizophrenic patients, postulating that it could diminish their hallucinations or cause them to function more effectively. In 1949 a European scientist, Nick Bercel, took LSD one time in Basel and discussed the effects of the substance with Carl Jung. Jung was fascinated by the many archetypes and other symbolic visions that LSD users reported anecdotally, although there is no suggestion that Jung himself ever experienced LSD. In the following decade and a half before LSD was made illegal, clinical researchers in Europe and the United States held some half dozen international conferences on the psychotherapeutic uses of psychedelics, published a handful of books on the subject, and produced no fewer than a thousand papers that documented the experiences of forty thousand subjects (Grinspoon and Bakalar 1997).

By the time Oscar Janiger undertook his monumental LSD study in 1954, pursuit of a diverse agenda for LSD research was well underway in Europe and North America. Scientists were investigating how the chemical worked, how it might impact alcoholics, and its potential role in effecting change in psychotherapy. Some were interested in exploring individuals' metabolic systems by observing how the body processed the substance. Other researchers hoped to use LSD to gain new insight into the nature and treatment of mental illnesses. Some 90 percent of European LSD researchers sought to discover the origins of schizophrenia, while others were interested in revealing how the mind works. One program used LSD to train psychiatric nurses and technicians at a hospital by giving the clinical staff LSD to facilitate understanding of the inner world of the mental health patients. In Czechoslovakia, it was believed that LSD could cut down psychotherapy time by a magnitude of ten to one. This was important in an era when psychoanalysis, generally requiring many sessions and even years of treatment, was the major technique employed to resolve psychotherapeutic issues. By the time Janiger became interested in the substance, perhaps as many as twenty researchers in the Los Angeles area were engaged in scientific studies utilizing LSD.

In the late 1950s and early 1960s the U.S. military, too, was interested in LSD. This was chronicled by the book *Acid Dreams*. In 1959 the *Wall Street Journal* wrote that hallucinogens, as they were being called by scientists, offered intriguing possibilities in the world of cloak-and-dagger counterespionage and perhaps on the battlefield as well. However, the combination of LSD's unreliability as a "truth serum" and the clear memories subjects retained of their LSD experiences made the substance all but useless for espionage purposes, and the military ceased research in 1963 (Lee and Shlain 1985).

The original hope that LSD would shed light on severe mental disorders like schizophrenia also received a setback when some early studies showed that schizophrenic patients, given LSD, felt alienated by the visions LSD produced and reported that these were different from their own hallucinations. Moreover, some researchers as early as 1952 believed that LSD was too uncontrollable a substance for psychotherapy, a conclusion that may have been directly related to the decision to conduct experiments in hospital rooms, where sensory deprivation was very much in evidence—white walls, white floors, white ceilings. Nonetheless, by the late 1950s a contingent of therapists both in the United States and abroad was reporting encouraging results in treating a variety of patients with LSD.

THE EFFECTS OF LSD: DESCRIBING THE INDESCRIBABLE

A detailed description of the LSD experience may help to illustrate why this substance generated so much interest among psychiatrists and researchers. Janiger documented four phases of the action of LSD. The first stage is distinguished, usually during the first hour, by the onset of physical changes that persist with some modification through the height of the experience. The second, or predominantly psychological, phase is ushered in with changes in visual perception, and lasts from one to five hours. The third period sees a gradual diminution of both the physical and psychological effects. Aftereffects that last one or more days constitute the final stage.

Typically, a person given a moderate oral dose of 100 mcg. of LSD begins to feel the effects about thirty minutes to one hour later. The person may become aware of some disconcerting physical signs, such as trembling, chills, feverishness, mild nausea, labored breathing, a feeling of intoxication, lethargy or a sense of tension, anxiety or expectancy. Often accompanying these are a decided emotional enhancement and lability. Commonly observed are overwhelming impulses to giggle or laugh, or, more rarely, to cry.

The physical effects in many individuals include marked fluctuations in blood pressure, pulse, respiration, body temperature, and pupilary and vasomotor functions. People who are fearful and anxious or strongly resistant and defensive with regard to the psychological changes caused by LSD can exhibit marked divergence in their autonomic nervous system response. Different reactions that people have under LSD range from extreme agitation, pacing, and flexing of muscles to relative immobility and catatonic-like states. Most of the people who took LSD in the Janiger project showed an inclination to lie down or remain passively seated whenever possible.

There may be frequent occurrence of generalized or specific pains at almost any site in the body. Some of Janiger's participants reported sensations of being crushed, drawn, pummeled, stretched, twisted, or squeezed. These descriptions may be symbolic expressions or may accurately diagnose reactions by susceptible tissues.

The second LSD stage documented by Janiger is characterized by changes in consciousness, attention and concentration, and intellectual functioning and suggestibility. Perceptual alterations are expressed by descriptions of visual hallucinations, pulsating and flowing movements, intensification of color, time distortion, and synesthesias. (Synesthesia is a process in which one type of stimulus produces a secondary subjective sensation. An example would be when a color evokes a specific smell.) Modifications in body image and self-concept are depicted together with feelings of depersonalization and detachment. The transcendental feelings of awe, illumination, profundity, sublimity, and affirmation are represented along with negative ideas of reference (an individual believes that others are targeting him or her for focus of attention or danger), paranoid delusions, and expressions of rage and self-destruction. Janiger's volunteers reported that their ability to recall events was heightened. Other frequently noted psychological phenomena include the alternating wavelike quality of the action of LSD, spatial distortions, and lightning shifts in a person's frame of reference.

The waning of such intense psychic experiences initiates the third stage of diminishing effects. Recovery, the fourth stage, may be accompanied by extreme exhaustion or renewed energy. Heightened sensitivity and awareness usually persist for some days. Most notably, Janiger's volunteers consistently reported crystalline recall of their inebriated states.

Dr. Janiger crafted a highly personalized composite picture of the essence of the LSD stages described above, gathering his material from several articulate and representative volunteer reports. He believed that the supremely individual nature of the drug experience best lent itself to this subjective form of presentation.

After you have become more familiar with the restless state of your nervous system, you settle down to wait for what will come. In about one hour, you begin to notice an extraordinary change in your state of consciousness. At first you seem rather confused, according to common sense standards. People ask you questions and you answer dreamily. You often feel that things are extraordinarily clear. You become alert and very sensitive to minute changes. You say: "I see! Now I begin to see," awed by revelation. Or if you are writing down your thoughts, you are reduced to translating the material of consciousness, which you cannot put into words, into mutilated metaphors or familiar analogies to describe that blinding clarity. You find that it has no counterpart in ordinary clear sensorium fed only by the trickles of common sense. Later, looking back from normal, less dilated consciousness, you remember that during the entire experience, you suspend ordinary logic without missing it. You felt given a refreshing rest. You enchant yourself with the airy thought that the experience has an odd logic of its own but it is quite enough to let it flood your brain and leave the question of whether your consciousness is clear or clouded to others.

Now your senses seem to take in more sight and sound. The eye becomes a camera with an automatic zooming lens. It rushes up for close, almost microscopic vision. And then your eye sends you strange messages that make you wonder: What if everything's alive? You see an animistic world living, walls inhaling, oil painting with muscles moving under the canvas. You endow these animated things with a conscious personality. You see the hedge breathing. It swells and subsides with a regular inhalation and expulsion of breath, calmly, contentedly. And suddenly you feel involved with life everywhere. You can't even light a cigarette in a detached way. Your perceptions are stretched before you can adjust to any illusions you have been seeing. You may feel ravenously hungry but your appetite is taken away or distracted by the birds outside singing to derange your senses. The sounds you should hear, you begin to see and touch, as if all your senses were on a single antenna. You can touch the sound, and watch it conduct the tempo of the breathing walls. You move your hand to the music and are moved to speak aloud. You stop, astonished, for your gesturing hand is entangled with your words. The words became a gesture, gestures graceful and gradual. Now wherever your eye falls on the resplendent world it seems to be a feast of the senses. You swear that you have seen the most beautiful sight ever seen by anyone on earth or anywhere. But you say this again of other signs. The color fantasies flow with great plasticity. The designs were formal, symmetrical and exquisitely perfect but drawn in jeweled illumined colors like melted precious stones. They formed patterns, which dissolved swiftly to be replaced by other patterns, scintillating transparencies, like filaments of amethysts and emeralds. And the light from within shines with such luminosity that you become overwhelmed by the beauty.

As you watch this show, you may lose all track of time. A new vista opens up all in a moment and while you feast upon it, time stands still. You have a feeling of nowness. There is no past or future. This moment, this ecstasy, is the only time you are alive. Happiness is not something to be experienced sometime in the future on vacation or after retirement. It is now. You are so aware of this precious moment, you feel it will pass. You make the sad comment on time's revenge. Time would pass and it would all end. In one of those minutes, an infinity of extraordinary events, lives and stories could be going on. Clock time is irrelevant. You are involved in a larger cosmic time, which tells you that in a flash you can see all.

Your mind may be flooded with all these vibrations, visions and flaming jewels, so that you may not be able to handle simple abstractions. You not only couldn't tell time, you may not concentrate on any assignment. Suddenly the meaning of the universe becomes completely clear, but you cannot make meaning from a proverb. It is a small insignificant question when you are synthesizing all the great paradoxes of cosmology. You begin to lose your inhibitions but you feel no compulsion to do anything bizarre. You don't want to be distracted but you are compliant. Someone asks what kind of music you would like to hear. You answer that it really makes no difference at all. Who has ten symphonies of colored chords detonating in his head? You can be moved around without interrupting your view of the visions—for you are the cameraman, director and projectionist and can show them where you please.

Of all the big changes you notice, the change in self-concept and body image is most immense. You feel at first no definite sharp location of yourself. This you, which stands outside yourself, shows no rigid shape. You feel dissociated and removed. Things, yourself, feel strange. You may see yourself writ large. You suddenly find yourself about fifteen feet tall looking down at your feet, which seem a long way away. You may take new pleasure in your body as if just discovering it. You may have a strange reaction to the mirror as if seeing a stranger. You feel able to step out of the rented costume of the self you held rigidly within narrow bounds.

When the visions are flowing, you actually see the things you describe. But when transcendent feelings flow, you want to describe unity, illumination, revelation, rebirth and exaltation. Then you are reduced to finding the most fantastic phrases to evoke the nonevocable. It is as if you saw a new color, one outside the band of the spectrum people normally see. You would need to use old words in wild ways. Or invent a new word, which communicates only to those who have seen your new color. It didn't come to you via logic but through direct contact, as if it sprouted within you in a class by itself. The world seemed right. LSD brings out a feeling of warmth, goodness, love, benevolence, laughter, great grinning at everything as if my personality were a Cheshire cat, all disappeared except this uncontaminated smile. This love may be what leads you to feel a sense of union.

At the very summit of the drug's effects, there is a feeling of continuum, of flowing. You feel as if we are, as individuals, no more than whirlpools in a river, but whirlpools with wills which can come together and join as one or disappear and join the river.

LSD may magnify defense and destructive impulses of which you're unaware. Like a lens, the drug blows them up to immense proportions. You may seek heaven with your reasoning mind and court hell with your heart. You may suffer from a rage to kill, have thoughts of suicide or believe you're being persecuted. You may feel that your friends are plotting against you, that everyone is watching you. You may move into jealousy. You may be suspicious that someone is going to take something of yours. You may believe that you are being deliberately poisoned. You may see an entire conspiracy. You may see no bright breathing jaws of fire, no divisions of dazzling splendor. The world may be drab and dead when not positively creeping with fearful plots and conspiracies. One [of the volunteers] wrote: "the whole experiment had been hell. There were no clear impressions of anything except pain and I wanted it to end. I said over and over again, 'I can't go through it. I can't.' It came to me that I had stopped life in my childhood, stopped living and merely been existing the rest of my life."

During the first experience, you do not care to bother with summoning spirits from the vast depths of your memory. You would rather watch the wild colors of the pageantry. You feel you would rather apply the Niagara of ideas flooding your brain to look into present problems. But you can turn and explore this flood of insights into the past. You may have a vision which resurrects in great detail an actual scene from childhood.

From the above description, which primarily depicts the second, psychological, stage of the LSD experience, it should be easy to imagine why LSD elicited such an enthusiastic response from psychologists. Especially when we consider that LSD is some five to ten thousand times more potent than another psychedelic, mescaline, it is not difficult to understand why LSD came to be so widely researched in this early period as an agent in psychotherapy, as a teaching and training aid in the psychiatric field, as a diagnostic device, as a method of investigating the creative, assimilative, and transcendental attributes of the mind, and as an unprecedented means to study psychic functioning (Hofmann 1980). It is ironic, overall, that the attention of the scientific world since the 1960s was primarily drawn to the aberrant and pathological nature of the drug's activity.

CLOSING THE DOORS OF PERCEPTION

Scientific research, both nationally and internationally, did come to an end. In 1962 legislation was passed that made research virtually impossible in the United States. Three years later the 1965 Drug Abuse Control Amendments made illicit manufacture and sale of LSD a misdemeanor. Then, in 1968, a bill was passed that made LSD sales a felony, and in 1970 regulations placed LSD in the Schedule 1 class (as a drug of abuse with no medicinal value). European research was also stilled, although some research has been conducted there in the last forty years. More importantly, it seems clear that social and media pressure, rather than scientific findings, directed the force of legislation. Early researchers of LSD, like Grof, continued to publish and search out alternate ways to alter conscious awareness, such as holotropic breathing. In Europe there have been recent moves to reopen research in this area.

Dr. Janiger was an early proponent of utilizing LSD in psychotherapy. In a paper published in 1959 in the *California Clinician,* he asserted that complications could be prevented by using precautions in screening prospective candidates for LSD-based treatments. If experienced psychotherapists were present, if patients were monitored in suitable surroundings, and if antidotes were readily available, he argued, the likelihood of having a safe procedure was excellent. Janiger wrote: "In our search for an unprecedented attack on the problems of self-understanding, we should welcome the help of a drug that truly enables us to heed the Talmudic injunction: we do not see things as they are, we see them as *we* are."

2

JANIGER'S REMARKABLE EXPERIMENT

BORN IN 1917, Janiger grew up on a small farm in upstate New York, but spent his student years in New York City, where he studied both humanities and sciences. As a Columbia University undergraduate who was interested from the start in a career in research, he heard accounts of plants that caused changes in consciousness and found himself fascinated by the botany of psychedelic plants. Consequently, his molecular biology studies were as much involved with plants as with human beings. He was also very interested in related information presented by early explorers.

Drawn to psychiatry after he obtained his medical degree from the University of California at Irvine, Janiger became one of the university's early research professors. From 1949 to the week before he died, he maintained a private psychiatric practice. In the early years he had an office in Los Angeles, worked hard, married his first wife, Helen, and kept very busy seeing patients and teaching classes at the California College of Medicine. Nonetheless, as early as 1954, he began to look around for a research program in which to involve himself.

Janiger had long been extremely interested in changes in consciousness, why and how these changes occurred, and what parts of the brain were involved. In particular he was drawn to the phenomenon of hallucinations. As a psychiatrist he heard about aberrant psychological states on a daily basis, especially among those of his patients who were psychotic. In 1953 Aldous Huxley published *Doors of Perception,* describing that author's experiences with hallucinogens, and Janiger was significantly influenced. The following year he began his landmark study of LSD effects.

As chapter 1 makes clear, Janiger was certainly not alone in his professional interest in LSD, and clinical research at the time was legal, encouraged, and, if not entirely respectable, at least not stigmatized. The corporate world provided much of the impetus and support for this research. Pharmaceutical companies with serendipitous discoveries, such as that of LSD, felt obliged to find some practical, medical use of the substance to justify their research and development budgets. The synthesizer of LSD-25, Sandoz Corporation, for example, encouraged physicians around the world to use LSD in clinical practice in the hopes of finding some true cure or treatment for illness. Janiger's timing was perfect.

THE STUDY'S ORIGINS

Despite his sustained interest in hallucinogenic substances, it was not until the early 1950s that Janiger, then thirty-five years old, first heard of LSD while teaching a class in general psychiatry at the California College of Medicine. As he spoke of substances that were used in various cultures to bring about different states of mind, such as the Navaho medicine peyote, Janiger mentioned his interest in botany and those plants that produced strange and untoward psychic experiences, and he reviewed the small but exciting and exotic literature that existed on the topic. One day a student brought along a friend to class, a young man named Bevins, who had heard of an unusual substance in Europe called LSD. He offered Janiger a sample of this material. At his home in Lake Arrowhead on a winter's day Janiger took the clear fluid, and over the next few hours had an astonishing experience. He thought that he wouldn't rest until he understood it as fully as he was able. He was as good as his word, and he spent the next fifty years looking at this substance and wondering what to do with it.

During this early period, Janiger became familiar with researchers involved in investigating altered states of consciousness and became friends with other people who worked with LSD. Some were very intelligent, progressive, and far-thinking visionaries. The scientific literature on LSD was growing. Janiger decided to call the Sandoz Corporation, the only company producing the substance, to determine the requirements for undertaking a project to investigate LSD's clinical effects. After a few weeks of negotiation with Sandoz, they were ready to start.

As mentioned previously, Sandoz was eager to find some medical use for the substance, and did not charge physicians to use it. Over the years the actual value of the LSD given to Janiger without cost represented a good deal of money. It would be almost impossible to set a price on it, however, since no market for LSD existed at the time. From a research-and-development perspective, Sandoz simply wanted to recoup its investment. Janiger was employed at the time by the University of California at Irvine, which provided him a research faculty affiliation. During the research period, however, Janiger paid his own rent on the Los Angeles house where the study was conducted as well as his staff's salary. He was allowed by Sandoz to charge a twenty-five-dollar administrative fee per client to help defray costs.

Janiger had a contact person in San Francisco for obtaining supplies of the drug from Sandoz. He would place an order, and the LSD would simply be mailed or delivered to his office. Over the years, this person was also very helpful in referring Janiger to professional articles on LSD research published in Europe and elsewhere. Janiger himself published very little on his research because most of his data fell into the category of phenomenological studies, which many of his peers did not consider particularly scientific.

Janiger planned his investigation as a large, naturalistic study of the phenomenological effects of LSD in human beings. He wanted to discover and report what LSD does if you just let it happen with appropriate safeguards in place. He proposed to minimize the amount of interference from the outside to avoid influencing participants, and he expressly did not want to program the volunteers to have any particular type of experience—not religious, spiritual, therapeutic, or creative.

Instead he sought to use a nondirected approach in an effort to identify the essential nature of the subjective state of the LSD experience, rather than to focus on any specific content reported by individual volunteers. To accomplish this, he designed a continuous data-gathering operation, with introductory interviews, progressive tape recordings, reports, and follow-up questionnaires; he cast his net widely to include a very large number of subjects; and he designed his study setting very carefully.

SET AND SETTING: A NATURALISTIC APPROACH

Janiger recognized early on the importance of participants' "set" (their mind-set at the time of the experiment) and study setting. To minimize the chance that his volunteers' set would undermine his attempt to discover LSD's characteristic effects, Janiger decided to gather a wide sample of normal, functioning volunteers who would be given graded doses of LSD in a uniform setting. The first group was basically drop-ins, friends of individuals who had been given LSD on a previous date. Hundreds of people showed up, offering themselves as subjects. Some were clients of Janiger and his colleagues, some were students, and some were friends of the above. There were older people, ministers, rabbis and priests, and one nun. Then there were the notables—the movie stars and the rich. By early 1962, when the initial phase ended, almost 930 persons had participated in the experience.

Candidates were selected from a large number of applicants who learned of the project first through word-of-mouth referral and, later, through public and professional notice. Initially, two broad groups of participants were involved: those in psychotherapy at the time (and designated as patients) and a cross-section of the general population. Enough volunteers were available to make possible a representative distribution of people by age, sex, religion, occupation, education, and diagnostic category. As the study progressed, a special group of professional artists were included. Gross personality disturbances or obvious health problems were ruled out through an initial interview with prospective volunteers. Chapter 3 details the volunteers' profiles.

To further minimize the chance that study results would be influenced by participants' mind-sets, a special effort was made not to "load the dice" by cueing the volunteers. They were told only that the experience would be a very powerful one for them, and monitors during their LSD experiences were reassuring but sparing with any suggestions. The volunteers were also told that if they wanted to end the experience, they would be able to do so at any time. Janiger believed that there was no real danger, and that proved to be the case.

During the first few years of the experiment, volunteers came to their sessions with almost no expectations about the presumed action of LSD. Janiger, of course, provided no indoctrination, and general information about the substance was virtually nonexistent. Toward the end of the 1950s, however, some information about LSD was being publicized. Consequently, later participants may have brought greater expectation of certain effects than did earlier volunteers, but there is no way to measure this. Certainly, there was little TV or media coverage. Public knowledge about LSD spread primarily by word of mouth in the Southern California area, as we see from the far-flung communities in the Los Angeles basin from which volunteers came—including Orange County, the San Fernando Valley, and Riverside County.

In addition to the attention he paid to volunteers' individual mindsets, Janiger also sought to create a setting that would minimally influence his study's outcomes. It was important to him that he interject as little of himself into the research as possible, and he decided that a natural setting would best facilitate his research goals. To the best of his knowledge, no prior studies had taken place in a naturalistic environment. In the beginning, however, he was not sure whether the pleasant setting was a contaminant, and he was wary of allowing music or pictures on the walls. He argued with colleagues endlessly about whether they should introduce anything that might be a bias. But Janiger understood also that the typical research setting, in which people were put in sterile rooms with white walls and enamel hospital beds, introduced a bias as well. Ultimately, Janiger concluded one could not conduct any study in a vacuum, nor eliminate all external influences. He decided to keep his set and setting as consistent as possible so that, at the very least, they would remain standard.

Janiger rented a small house on Wilton Place in Los Angeles that had once belonged to the silent film star Clara Bow for the duration, and used part of the house for his psychiatric practice and the rest for the research. There was a pleasant living room, a garden, and several smaller rooms ideal for conducting the type of experiment he had in mind. Shortly after the study began, one room was outfitted as an artist's studio with facilities for painting, drawing or sculpting. The neighborhood was quiet and pleasant.

In the living room a sofa was set up, and there was a cot for lying down. There were paintings on the wall and bric-a-brac scattered about. Assorted records were available for the volunteers, and their particular preferences, if any, were noted. Some preferred tranquil Mozart, water sounds, or sounds of nature, while others wanted modest percussion or opera. Some wanted nothing at all. No one insisted that any particular music be played. Maintaining the volunteer's comfort level while they were under the influence of LSD was the primary concern.

The great majority of volunteers had their experiences inside the Wilton house. However, occasionally someone would want to or be encouraged to go outside, either to the garden or to a coffee shop with a monitor. Participants never left the Wilton Place house by themselves. In all cases the individuals did what they wanted to do. Occasional departures from standard procedure occurred when some participants took LSD at two other houses Janiger owned or when other psychologists brought their clients to Janiger for LSD doses but then left with the clients in tow.

Janiger chose to be inductive in his research, without fixed ideas, to follow along with whatever the volunteers decided to do. He tried to keep the experiment totally open-ended, to take a natural history approach to the psychedelic, allowing the experience to speak for itself. The metaphor that he used for his method was to see how he could keep the boat going along with as light a hand as possible on the tiller.

JANIGER'S METHOD(S)

Working with more than 930 people was indeed a challenge. That is, 930 different days of Janiger's life were given over to monitoring the well-being of the volunteers. He carefully screened them all, checking to be sure no one suffered from psychosis. He ruled out severe physical and mental disorders, such as heart and liver disease, kidney disorders, schizophrenia, and gross personality disturbances. All volunteers were given a mental status exam to ensure that they were alert and oriented in time and place. Volunteers were asked about prior hospitalization, serious illnesses, and ongoing psychotherapy. All were asked if they had ever taken LSD or other mind-altering substances before. Janiger was the only person who screened the volunteers, and he sent away anyone who had clear health problems or neurotic or psychotic features.

Following the screening process participants were told to report in the morning after having a minimal breakfast. Janiger generally had a nurse or nurse-intern on hand. At about 8:00 A.M. LSD was given orally on the basis of two micrograms per kilogram of body weight, which was considered a moderate dose by midcentury psychotherapeutic standards. In this way, a 150 lb. (68 kg.) man would be given 136 mcg. of LSD. (By way of comparison, street doses of LSD today generally range from 60 to 80 mcg.) Each person was carefully monitored during the active LSD experience, and observations were made about general behavior.

Janiger tended toward conservative doses when administering LSD. However, in one study, he gave a high dose of 2,000 to 3,000 mcg. to a professor from one of the medical schools in Northern California, who had shown very remarkable control with normal low doses. The professor was a ski trooper during World War II and was a vigorous, healthy man. He did fine with the high dosage, reporting simply that he reached a place where everything was whitened out and that he went in and out of conscious awareness over a period of several hours. He reported no special effects from the experience, however. In another case Janiger administered a 1,000-mcg. dose to a participant who volunteered to undergo tooth extraction without pain medication. To the dentist's astonishment, the dose worked as a dissociative anesthetic, and the extraction was performed painlessly.

In those early days of psychedelic research, there were no university institutional review boards and no particular protocols to follow. A brief physical examination was conducted prior to the administration of the LSD. The volunteer was then given an informational sheet to fill out and asked to sign an informed consent form. The form was dated and witnessed by a second person. It read as follows:

I request that LSD be given to me for experimental purposes. The nature of this medication and its possible dangers and consequences have been explained to me in full, and I understand them thoroughly.

I accept the responsibility for any complications that may arise during or following this experiment that is being given at my request.

The LSD from Sandoz was pure, without any street additives, and, thus, reasonably safe. Generally, no one would be under the effects of LSD without a second person present in the room as monitor, although that person would not necessarily interact with the volunteer. On occasion the monitor would be in the outside waiting room, a few feet away. Only on two occasions were the experiences overwhelming for the volunteers, necessitating the administration of a tranquilizer.

The degree of mobility varied among the participants. Many lay quietly on the cot to attend to their internal experiences, some using blinkers to keep out the daylight. Others walked about the house. A number went to a coffee shop down the street, accompanied by a monitor. A permissive atmosphere prevailed, with few restrictions on peoples' behavior. Most participants did not eat during the height of the experience, which lasted between four and five hours from the time they ingested the LSD. The effects lasted most of the day, and by evening the volunteers would be finished. Advance arrangements were made for participants to be accompanied home by someone responsible when the experience ended, and they were advised to remain in contact with Janiger for several days following.

In keeping with Janiger's data-gathering system, each person was asked to make notes and write a detailed report of the experience as soon as possible, usually at the end of the day. Many volunteers attempted to write during the LSD experience itself, a project fraught with difficulty, as we will see in their reports in subsequent chapters. Volunteers then systematically analyzed their narratives using a method known as Q-sorting to generate data Janiger would later use to identify core characteristics of the LSD experience. We will look at some of these reports and the results of the Q-sort in chapter 3. Additionally, Janiger believed that it was important to conduct some kind of follow-up with volunteers to determine the effects of the LSD on their lives and well-being. Thus, thirty days after volunteers had received their LSD doses, they were sent a comprehensive questionnaire in the mail (See appendix I). About 70 percent of the volunteers returned their questionnaires. A more comprehensive follow-up was funded and completed in 1998 by the Multidisciplinary Association for Psychedelic Studies (MAPS). For the most part, results from the follow-ups were very positive, and we will look at that material in chapter 4.

As the experiment progressed, Janiger developed a number of sub-projects. These included a study to be described (in chapter 3) of two identical twins, young women whose lives were very much entangled prior to their LSD experiences and quite individualistic after. Another special project dealt with a fireman who was quite socially inhibited and repressed but of average intelligence. He was given 25 mcg. of LSD periodically over an entire year and eventually became an extrovert, much to the surprise of his coworkers. A third small sub-study investigated LSD's potential to block pain (the tooth extraction mentioned previously was part of this experiment), another observed people's capacity to work as a group under the influence of LSD, and yet another sought to block LSD's effects.

The largest substudy involved artists, who got wind of the experiment early on and came in great numbers to paint or sketch under the influence of LSD. The project began when an artist became very excited by a Hopi kachina doll that Janiger happened to have in his office. The artist insisted that he sketch it during his LSD experience, and said afterward that one LSD experience was like a four-year course in art school. Consequently, so many artists volunteered that Janiger designed the separate artists' project to keep them from skewing the demographics of his general study population. A room was set aside as an art studio and equipped with an easel, pens, pencils, oils, and sculpting tools. Typically, the artists were asked to render the kachina doll in their usual style prior to taking the LSD. Then, an hour or so into the LSD experience, they would be asked to render the same doll a second time. Much more will be said about this study in chapter 5.

STUDY'S END

The LSD project proceeded for eight years. As word got out about the study, more and more people asked to be included. Janiger's files are, in fact, full of letters from individuals who knew others who were involved in or aware of the study, and who wanted to participate. Janiger was satisfied with the progress of the research, and he convinced Sandoz Corporation officials to allow him to continue as the numbers of volunteers kept increasing. Janiger's hope was to be able to get a clean thousand participants by study's end.

However, Janiger had realized from the first that a shutdown of the research would be inevitable. This awareness partially accounts for his research goal to gather as much information as possible over as wide a range of topics as possible, in order to gather preliminary data and impressions that would illuminate promising areas of research. He hoped that any promising leads could be explored in the future by others when the foreseeable reaction against psychedelics would have run its course. His approach was like the fox rather than the hedgehog, in that he chose to explore a wide terrain rather than burrow down deep in one area. He thought he could provide a jump start to a myriad of subsequent studies.

Until 1962 the sole supply of LSD was in the hands of researchers. There were virtually no nonmedical sources of the drug available in the United States prior to that date, and only a small number of physicians were involved in LSD research. However, a reservoir of elite users gradually accumulated, turned on by researchers but subsequently without access to the drug they had grown to like. Illicit LSD began to be made and was first synthesized in California in 1962. By the end of Janiger's research in mid-1962, the psychedelic era in America was taking off like wildfire. Like an S curve in investment theory, the phenomenon of psychedelic use came into U.S. and European societies slowly, then picked up speed and took off.

By 1963 Timothy Leary and Richard Alpert were expelled from Harvard because of their freewheeling advocacy of LSD. Articles about LSD appeared in the mass media, opening the door to everyone who had not yet heard of it. By 1964 use of black-market LSD, often mixed with other substances, was widespread. In 1965 California made LSD illegal except in the hands of authorized investigators. As mentioned in chapter 1, the federal government passed stiff legislation in 1966 prohibiting the use of LSD. In the popular mind LSD had become the scapegoat for many tragedies that it may not have caused. One in particular was a hoax purporting that a group of youth under the effects of LSD stared at the sun until it blinded them. As we saw in the introduction, the effect of these developments was to extinguish the promise of Janiger's study, and the reactions against LSD research would persist up to the turn of the twenty-first century.

RESULTS AND CONCLUSIONS

During the eight years of the Wilton Place study a rich and fascinating range of personal accounts of the LSD experience filled Janiger's file cabinets. Many originated from the psychotherapy patients and artists, who were overwhelmingly enthusiastic about their LSD experiences. Janiger was surprised to learn that LSD provided a substantial learning curve, with many artists becoming more adept each time they worked under the influence of the drug. Artists somehow found a way to harness the LSD state to the creation of art and were able increasingly to control the physical expression of their subjective experiences. The files also held reports from some dozen luminaries, including some of Hollywood's top writers. One notable, Clark Gable, gave an interview to a local Florida newspaper about his psychological breakthroughs from LSD, but for the most part these files remain locked away because of psychiatric privilege in law, which belongs to the client.

Janiger didn't report any critically negative effects on volunteers. Contrary to often sensationalized reports in the contemporary media, he observed no psychotic episodes. No one was hospitalized because of traumatic effects, although there are many reports of severe physical pain and anxiety. There were only two occasions when it was necessary for Janiger to intervene because he had reason to fear that a volunteer was going to hurt himself. Working out the figures, only .002 percent, or two thousandths, of volunteers had an untoward effect necessitating the use of thorazine to calm them or minimize the LSD effects. Only twenty-five people felt the LSD experience was stronger than they expected, or less pleasant, and more disturbing, than they had hoped.

Reflecting on the study in an interview with MAPS as they prepared to publish their forty-year follow-up, Janiger summarized his work. He explained that his purpose had been an attempt to define the nature of the LSD experience as a special state of consciousness. Thus the LSD experience would be seen as a different consciousness state, such as sleep, wakefulness, hypnotic trance, and the like.

His research demonstrated that the world according to LSD is an idiosyncratic one. The nature of the individual drug experience reflects the basic psychophysiological action of the substance as it interacts with the total life experience that the person brings to it. Understanding the relative contributions that are made by the drug or by the individual was, for Janiger, a fascinating and formidable challenge, like attempting to distinguish a dream from the dreamer. As his understanding of the experience grew, he concluded that LSD does not necessarily favor any particular psychotherapeutic model or mystical or spiritual belief, nor did it necessarily fit any specific group of systematized ideas. Rather, it seemed to produce a marked shift in our fundamental perceptual frame of reference upon which humans' ongoing concept of reality rests. Such a change in our habitual way of being in the world can lead to a profound psychic shake-up, providing startling insights into the nature of reality and into how our personal existence is fashioned.

Reflecting on the effects of the LSD research on his career, Janiger believed that—at the beginning—the research was professionally as well as personally rewarding. It certainly was interesting and gripping material to work with. Many other scientists asked him about his work, and several colleagues wanted to try the LSD themselves. After a period of time, Janiger came to be seen as something of a pariah, somehow marginal, as he continued his experimental studies and did not publish his results. However, there seem to have been no professional repercussions, and the research did not interfere with his medical career. He continued to maintain his academic position. During the entire period of the research, no negative experiences were linked to his research nor were any accusations lodged against him.

In 1986 Janiger returned to his early study and hosted an art show in his Santa Monica, California, home of the paintings and drawings artists generated during their LSD experiences. With author de Rios in 1989, he published an article in the *Journal of Psychoactive Drugs* called "LSD and Creativity." The paper analyzed the artwork created under LSD and set it in the context of its historical moment. More will be said about this in chapter 5.

3

(UN)CHARACTERISTICS OF THE LSD EXPERIENCE

JANIGER REALIZED that this new substance, LSD, that he had on hand was unlike anything else he had ever encountered. True, as he often recounted, the British used sodium pentathol, the so-called truth serum, in psychiatric practice to help speed up the psychotherapy process, but the LSD he now had available for study was in a class by itself. Deciding to cast a very wide net and to learn all he was able about this substance, Janiger was well in keeping with his sincere and profound interest in knowlege for its own sake. Unlike bench scientists with myopia-like approaches to research, a kind of a + b = c method, Janiger was always interested in synthesis and overviews—the larger picture. He realized that he would be able to answer his own questions about the substance by obtaining a large sample of volunteers and by simply persevering at this work.

In this chapter, we will examine the participants close-up, as well as their backgrounds, occupations, and expectations. As the study went along, Janiger hit upon a novel way to make sense of and synthesize the variety within the LSD experience, looking not only at the uniqueness of each person's experience, but also at the constants or regularities of effect among individuals. In the world of consciousness studies we run into the term *intersubjectivity* time and again. Since subjectivity is so very personal and private, how on earth could one person ever get inside the head of another and experience his or her particular experiences? Not an easy one, that! But Janiger was undaunted by the challenge. He settled on the use of a research technique, called a Q-sort, which enabled him to tap into many of the volunteers' private and personal experiences. We'll look at this technique as well. Finally, we will set the results of the volunteers' personal experiences with LSD within a more general framework of altered states of consciousness, proposed some years ago by the psychologist Arnold Ludwig.

THE STUDY PARTICIPANTS

As we learn more about the LSD volunteers, the reader is likely to note that the numbers of participants appears to keep changing. Over the eight-year period, the overload of seeing patients overwhelmed the structure set up by Janiger. Record keeping became somewhat chaotic after the 860th client. In Janiger's estimation, the final number of clients given LSD was around 930. Tallies and analysis were done on the first 667 participants, allowing us to report some interesting profiles. There were 409 men and 258 women involved in this early tally. Unfortunately, many data pages are incomplete. Two hundred fifty-six of those tallied were professional people, including doctors, lawyers, accountants, nurses, teachers, and college professors. Another 223 were in the building trades, or were housewives, secretaries, office, or factory workers. Musicians, artists, writers, actors, and media people represented another 118 participants.

The years and numbers of participants, too, are interesting to track. Unlike the illicit LSD users of the 1960s, who were mainly college age, members of the Janiger experiment were typically thirty to forty-five and from middle to upper socioeconomic levels. They had their LSD experience in an experimental or psychotherapy setting and were given LSD by a physician. The participants involved were not deviant in any way. Janiger wanted to know to what extent a reasonably mature and well-educated group of people would be attracted to the use of LSD, how and for what reasons they would use LSD, and what the net consequences would be after a number of years. This group of people provides us with information of vital social importance.

While the data on numbers are not complete, in 1956 only 5 people were given LSD. In 1957 the number rose to 22, then 100 people in 1958, 181 at the height of the experiment in 1959, 111 in 1960, 96 in 1961, and 74 in 1962. Thus we see that the fewest number of people clearly were at the beginning of the study, while a bell curve took shape as the experiment progressed, tapering off by 1962. Participants came from all over the Los Angeles basin and surrounding counties, as well as from San Francisco; San Diego; Miami Beach; Palm Springs; Seattle; New York; Cambridge, Massachusetts; Boulder, Colorado; Columbus, Ohio; Flint, Michigan; Saskatchewan; and France. There were 96 different job titles given by the participants. While ages ranged from eighteen to eighty-one, the average age of the participant was in the early thirties. Six subjects were under the age of twenty, while seven were over the age of sixty. Many of the referrals came from Janiger, but others were referred by psychological colleagues and former participants. Most of the volunteers were middle- and upper-middle-income men and women, although some 75 people ranked lower in income. A fair number of the people who were college graduates also had graduate degrees. One hundred forty-two had a high school education. A few completed only grade school.

Many different religious affiliations could be noted among the volunteers. These included 163 Christians—including 48 Catholics, 4 Baptists, 13 Unitarians, 9 Methodists, 4 Presbyterians, 5 Episcopalians, 1 Lutheran, 1 Congregationalist, and 78 people from other Protestant denominations. More than 150 individuals were of nonorganized religious affiliation. Many volunteers listed themselves as nonsectarian or agnostic. Eighty-one people were Jewish. There were 15 members of the Church of Religious Science, and 7 reported that they were members of Eastern religions. More than 100 people stated that they had no religion, and 9 stated that they were atheist.

Interestingly, 236 people stated that they had previously been in psychotherapy, despite the fact that the study was not oriented toward a clinical population. More than 100 people represented themselves as artists. Among the professional groups, there were 37 physicians and surgeons. Twenty-seven volunteers were psychotherapists, which included psychologists and psychiatrists. Twenty-seven were teachers. Eleven were professors of chemistry, psychology, pharmacology, art history, anthropology, zoology, world religions, and biochemistry. There were 4 ministers, 1 nun, 6 attorneys, 13 engineers, and 2 dentists.

Seven of the volunteers were social workers in the fields of rehabilitation and youth counseling or were state consultants or training advisors. There were 2 chiropractors as well. Eleven scientists included mathematicians, physicists, computer programmers, logistics specialists, communications/space technology workers, and postdoctoral researchers. Other professionals represented were philosophers, interns, a library administrator, a radio news analyst, nurses, a geologist, a translator, an ophthalmologist, and a hypnotist. Among business people were found salesmen, real estate brokers, storekeepers, accountants, a chain-store executive, and publishers and advertisers. Other businesspeople included an insurance claims adjuster, a florist, a beauty-shop owner, a jeweler, a model, secretaries, a clerk-typist, a hospital administrator, a theater administrator, a freight-rate clerk, a duplicating operator, a retired government clerk, and a madam (prostitute). There were business managers in sales, personnel, restaurants, banks, and offices. There were manufacturers of business materials, ladies' apparel, and office supplies. Three contractors in the electrical and building trades also volunteered. Among the 106 people in the artists group were painters, muralists, sculptors, writers, actors, musicians, and composers, a motion-picture producer, a movie director, a photographer, a stage designer and manager, a film editor, a cartoonist, and a singer. There were four civil servants, including a fireman, a deputy sheriff, a postal handler, and a parole agent. Additionally, there were laboratory technicians and 17 laborers, including mechanics, assemblers, waiters, gardeners, welders, a flight attendant, and a pressman.

When we look at the world of psychological research in general, it is important to note that most of the studies published in all fields of psychology utilize college sophomores as volunteers. What a contrast to Janiger's multilayered collection of men and women, who truly represent all walks of life. When we look at the many similarities that these distinctive individuals reported in their LSD experiences, we can see how valuable this study was in delineating the common characteristics of the LSD experience.

REASONS FOR VOLUNTEERING FOR THE LSD PROJECT

Now that we have a clear sense of the backgrounds and profiles of the LSD participants, let's examine the volunteers' stated reasons for participating in the experiment. There are almost as many reasons as there are participants, but at some point when 612 individuals had been queried, their explanations were codified by Janiger and his staff. Some volunteers sought insight into their behavior or to explore and clarify their personal problems. Others wanted relief from crippling inhibitions, such as perfectionism, critical acuity, or insecurity. Others wanted to have mystical experiences—to experience oneness with the universe—to enhance their creativity, or to become more sensitive as writers. Others wanted to expand their consciousness. Some wanted a deeper understanding of themselves and reality. Others wanted to find out who they really were and to gain insight, understanding, and purpose in life. A few wanted release from a long-held resentment against another person.

Some of the volunteers were curious to see how the LSD differed from another drug, such as mescaline or peyote. Others had a scientific interest and curiosity. A few wanted a new emotional and visual experience, more free visualization and response. Another wanted to find a reason for his stuttering. One writer wanted "chemical Christianity" to overcome spiritual poverty. Some wanted a deeper sense of place in relationship to others in the world. One woman wanted to be very happy. Another woman wanted to control her obesity. Several volunteers believed that LSD might help them with marital problems. One woman wanted to quit smoking. Another man had a desire to stop drinking. A man wanted to discover and recall significant traumatic formative experiences in his life. Another woman wanted spiritual enlightenment. Another wanted to gain insight into the creative process. A woman wanted to understand her fear of men. Another wanted to release memory blocks and emotional expression. One man had an interest in extrasensory perception.

THE LSD CONSTANTS

Janiger's main goal in the research was to discover and identify the essential characteristics of the LSD state as opposed to the widely varying and individualistic content that came into play. A useful analytic technique to tease out the essentials of this state involved a very simple Q-sort design. The first participant provided a written report of his own LSD experience. Based on that report Janiger created a series of index cards with descriptions from the report logged on the cards. In this way, all notable elements of that person's experience were transferred to a collection of cards. A similar process was conducted with the second volunteer, and new cards were created to describe any new experiences that the participants had reported. The next participant was then asked to review all the cards and sort them into three piles. The first pile was for descriptions of experiences that were identical to his or her own. The second pile was for descriptions that were somewhat similar to previous volunteers' experiences. The third pile was for descriptions that were not at all similar to what others had experienced. This process was reiterated time and time again. Unfortunately, we do not have an exact figure of how many times this occurred, but the number of Q-sort cards ran into the hundreds, and there were a remarkably small number of cards in the first pile that represented the common, identical experiences. Janiger then reviewed the Q-sort coding to delineate the LSD constants. Research protocols today would take a different tack. Most likely, two or more research assistants, knowing nothing of the project at hand, would conduct independent syntheses. Then a reliability statistic would be generated to see how close the "blind" researchers came to agreement, with no bias in sight. Janiger did not follow this protocol.

Janiger used only the data that he was given by the volunteers and that emerged naturally from their reports. As the project grew larger, the data became overwhelming and not all of it was analyzed. Unfortunately, the project was begun before computers were in widespread use. Nonetheless, and taking into consideration the incompleteness of his data, Janiger felt confident identifying the categories shown on page 33 as core characteristics of the LSD experience.

Clearly, given the large number of volunteers' comments on their experiences, analyzing the data was not an easy task. The volunteers worked from the prose of those individuals who preceded them, prose that was concrete and descriptive. Janiger had to abstract and generalize

CORE CHARACTERISTICS OF LSD YIELDED BY Q-SORT

Real, visual, and auditory hallucinations	Recall and reliving
Anxiety and fear	Alertness
Cramps, paralysis, and agony	Importance, purpose, meaning, real
Paranoid feelings	Appreciation, depersonalization, and natural vs. artificial
Depression, guilt, and irritation	
Somatic discomfort	Mystical
Strange body feelings	Relaxation and quiet
Dreamy and hypnogogic	Euphoria and laughter
Internal—visual images and synesthesia	Comparisons with drinking behavior
	Disappointed or no reaction
Perceptual distortions	Interpersonal relations
Inhibitions	Experiencing time
Confusion and mind flooded	Orgiastic
Attention, communication, short-term memory	Insightful/therapeutic
Unreality, newness, strangeness	Artistic and creative insight and appreciation

from this plethora of information to a somewhat more conceptual terminology. He tried to stay as close as possible to the actual wording of the volunteers when assigning category names to the Q-sort piles made by volunteers. Janiger considered the twenty-eight categories listed above to be *constants* of the LSD experience, that is, effects experienced by enough of his volunteers that he could consider them characteristic. Two additional categories, "the experience left me feeling" and "miscellaneous," are comprised of very diverse experiences, thus not constants as such. Rather, they group volunteers' experiences that did not fit into other categories, and show Janiger's strong desire to avoid distorting or misrepresenting the data. One might say that, in their diversity, these last two categories do suggest that idiosyncrasy is always a core characteristic of the LSD experience.

THE CONSTANTS IN CONTEXT: LUDWIG'S ANALYSIS OF ALTERED STATES OF CONSCIOUSNESS

From his Q-sort data Janiger delineated the above LSD constants. To put them in perspective, it is useful to place these characteristics of the LSD experience within the context of the broad range of experiences we refer to as altered states of consciousness. LSD-induced consciousness is just one type of altered mental state known to social scientists. Meditation, fasting, flagellation, hypnosis, trance phenomena induced by rhythmic dancing, musical chants, and other activities readily spring to mind as ways that people have changed their phenomenal reality throughout history. There is abundant anthropological evidence that human beings have long sought to experience altered mental states in order to find supernatural solace or direction, learn about their environment, and achieve social cohesion in society.

In 1969 psychologist Arnold Ludwig identified a series of ten general characteristics of altered states of consciousness, after analyzing existing reports in the scientific literature. We will now examine Janiger's data through the lens of Ludwig's model, identifying the features of the LSD experience that fit these universal categories, as well as those that do not. It is interesting to note that Janiger's work, which predated Ludwig's, was specifically data-driven, rather than of a secondary nature drawing upon other studies.

The following are Ludwig's ten general characteristics of altered states of consciousness:

1. **Alterations in Thinking.** At a subjective level, varying disturbances in concentration, attention, memory, and judgment occur, with a possible decrease in reflective awareness.
2. **Disturbed Time Sense.** The sense of time and chronology alters; people may feel a sense of timelessness, or time may be experienced as either slowing down or accelerating. Time may also seem to be infinite or unbelievably short in its duration.
3. **Loss of control.** People may show an initial fear of losing their grip on reality or else losing self-control. They may offer some resistance to experiencing an altered state of consciousness or

may willingly wish to enter this state, especially if they live in a society characterized by beliefs that they can experience divinity or become mouthpieces for a god or gods through such activity.

4. **Change in Emotional Expression.** People display emotional extremes ranging in degree from ecstasy and orgiastic equivalents to profound fear and depression.

5. **Changes in Perception of Body.** People frequently report various body-image distortions that refer to their perceived boundaries in space and their relationships with others. Some individuals experience a profound sense of depersonalization or a schism between body and mind. Others report a dissolution of the boundaries that separate themselves from others, the world, or the universe. These body changes are seen as strange and even frightening. People may report dizziness, vision blurring, numbness, and lack of pain.

6. **Perceptual Distortions.** There is increased visual imagery, hyperacuteness of perceptions, and illusions.

7. **Change in Life's Meaning or Significance.** Many people exhibit a strong tendency to attach special significance to experiences, ideas, or perceptions that develop while they are in an altered state. In the wake of such experiences people report great insight or profound feelings or meaning

8. **Sense of the Ineffable.** After experiencing such states people report a difficulty in communicating the nature of it to someone who is uninitiated. They find the experience to be too overwhelming to be expressed or described in words, although they don't hesitate to try to do so!

9. **Feelings of Rejuvenation.** In the wake of the experience often comes a new sense of hope, rejuvenation, or rebirth.

10. **Hypersuggestibility.** There is an increased likelihood that people will uncritically accept or respond to specific statements or nonspecific cues in order to seek support or guidance to relieve some of the anxiety associated with loss of control. Thus the suggestions of a person guiding the session may be wholly relied upon without reflection.

Now let's examine the relationship between Ludwig's characteristics of altered states and the common characteristics Janiger identified among the participants in his LSD study. The remarks in quotations are drawn from the actual wording on the Q-sort cards generated by the first 168 volunteers to best describe their own experiences.

Alterations in thinking, or more generally speaking, cognitive changes, are certainly evident in the words of the Janiger volunteers. The Q-sort yielded several categories that indicate distinct cognitive changes experienced by most of the study participants: confusion and mind flooding, attention, communication and short-term memory, and recall and reliving of an earlier experience. VR wrote: "I was completely aware of my realistic circumstances and my immediate surroundings. I could consciously report and discuss the most intensely bizarre hallucinations with people in the room where they were taking place. I had almost total recall." Another volunteer saw one animal pass imperceptibly into and reenter another animal; one long continuous chain of animals melting and merging and fusing into other animals. He wrote: "Lots of trembling. I was scared and I couldn't concentrate on anything." That same volunteer wrote that he was able to solve some materialistic problems, such as how to present himself and his ideas to certain persons in regard to a position that he wanted. Another wrote, "My contacts with others were so empathetic that I had this wonderful feeling of communicating with others that one enjoys only when he is communicating at all levels." Some self-reports are hilarious, like this one from a writer who wrote that he felt like Peter Pan in the laughing universe: "I felt that laughter was infinite. It was a separate permanent, everlasting state." Ten hours later, he wrote: "I looked for a pen, hoping I could remember enough physics to work on the formula for turning carbon and hydrogen into laughter."

The second of Ludwig's characteristics, a disturbed sense of time, is also widely reported among the study participants and was classified by Janiger simply as "experiencing time." Q-sort phrases included the following: "Everything comes in waves, pulsations, vibrations. Now seems forever. Time seems unimportant. I can change past events. Past, present and future are all together now. Time isn't. Falling objects seem to drift slowly to the floor. Time seemed to have come to a complete standstill.

Every minute seemed hours and time was dragging." One volunteer wrote: "Time often stood still. I'd look out the window and giggle, and seemingly 10 or 15 minutes later, I'd look again, and everything was exactly the same." Another volunteer wrote: "I was in a timeless world—timeless because whatever came to my attention became the subject of total experience."

The third universal identified by Ludwig, loss of control, was also widely experienced among the LSD volunteers. The Q-sort phrases illustrate: "Certain things are frightening me. I have some fear that I might become permanently insane. I'm afraid that I will tremble uncontrollably when I use my hands. I don't like letting loose of my hold on sanity this way. I seem to be on the fringes of sheer horror or fearful that something dreadful is about to happen. I'm caught in terror. I have never known such a complete and utter state of helplessness." One volunteer wrote: "My problem of expression and communication brought me to an experience of what I felt to be insanity. I pictured myself giggling grotesquely for everyone near me to see, while inside of me were locked up sane and reasonable thoughts. I said to myself, so this is the horror of the asylum. People who appear as idiots are all the while wanting to express themselves." Another volunteer wrote: "My tongue began to feel quite swollen. I felt that I was burning. My body was out of control. My legs wouldn't hold me up and I needed to lean on something."

Changes in emotional expression dominate volunteers' reports. The Q-sort categories that show these extremes include "Anxiety and Fear" and "Depression." While no named constant indicates it, there are positive emotional extremes represented in the constants and a significant number of people did report positive emotional extremes. One volunteer wrote: "I burst into tears and cried bitterly. Then my sadness vanished as I became completely absorbed in the petal of a rose which fell to the ground." Another volunteer, in a positive appraisal, wrote: "In the aftermath, I think this has been the most wonderful experience of my life. It is certainly the one in which I have experienced the world most intensely. The world has a touch of magic about it now. It is more real than it has ever seemed before."

Changes in perception of one's body, as observed in Ludwig's work, are ubiquitous in Janiger's reports. Some Q-sort phrases that indicate such shifts include the following: "My mouth is very dry. I have funny feelings on my skin. I feel weak. My left hand is real numb. My voice sounds different. One half of my body felt differently from the other half. Parts of my body don't seem to belong to me. The shape of my body doesn't seem normal. My body seems to be doing strange things all on its own, changing in size, growing younger or older. My hands and feet feel peculiar. I feel like I'm floating in space. I feel as if I am melting, disintegrating, turning into a liquid."

Ludwig's sixth constant, perceptual distortion, was one of the most difficult experiences for the volunteers, as they had not anticipated these sensory changes and often feared they were going crazy. Many had visual and auditory hallucinations, vivid scenes which seemed very real at the time. They saw and heard things happening which couldn't be so, yet seemed very real. The Q-sort phrases are illustrative: "The things I see out of nowhere seem like they're really there. I see faces of little animals coming out of the walls. I heard wonderful music playing but there wasn't any. People, some of whom I'd known in the past, others right out of thin air appear. Hallucinations of almost a cosmic nature. Help! Panic. I feel a sense of nameless terror all about me. I smell something that I know is not really there. Other peoples' faces seem to have become changing masks. My hearing seems sharper than usual. I seem to have developed X-ray vision. Walls seem to be breathing." One volunteer reported the following perceptual distortions: "I'm going in and out of temperature changes that are so abrupt. Temperature changes were also in color—like passing through vertical bands of color. Cold was always the intense blue. The blue became everything. Oh God. Did I have a color of crying? Oh God this is beautiful. The color of crying was like a shimmering curtain of sparkly things. The color varied. Mostly pearl and alabaster. The feeling was that blue . . . blue . . . like it was lit with fire but it was blue."

Realizing a change in life's meaning or significance characterized many volunteers' experiences. The Q-sort phrases frequently indicated that people came to understand things far differently than before. They reported feeling much more creative. Some saw wasted effort in life. A shift in values from material to nonmaterial often occurred. Their comments included the following: "The most important things in the world right now are my thoughts. Everything seems to have a symbolic meaning in it. Only now do I really see the point of existence. Objects seem more real. I seem to be seeing myself as I am." One volunteer wrote: "I value LSD primarily as an extraordinarily effective releasing agent. I continue to experience a residual feeling of release, exhilaration and extended perception. I am curious and responsive to all phases of nature."

Ludwig's sense of the ineffable, too, was typical as volunteers reported having trouble expressing themselves. The Q-sorts describe this paradox of feeling that words cannot possibly suffice, but then the volunteers go on to describe their experiences in illustrious detail. "Words are inadequate. Everything is inter-related with everything else in a way which ordinarily wouldn't seem possible. There is no such thing as cause and effect, everything just happens of its own accord. I can see all the mysteries of the universe in a single leaf. Opposites seem to be related in a strange paradoxical way. There seems to be a pattern inherent in everything. A sense of deeper understanding of love and hate, good and bad. This was the true meaning of eternity. I felt on the verge of some Great Understanding, that with a little straining, I could have the explanation for everything." One volunteer wrote: "A trip to never-never land. It is impossible to adequately describe the experience in words. It is the LSD which induces these utterly unbelievably fantastic changes in the human mind. If you can imagine yourself wide awake in the most beautiful dream world, [t]hat's LSD."

Feelings of rejuvenation were widespread in the reports. Q-sort statements reflect a sense of rebirth and optimism: "The physical symptoms I had when I came in seemed to have cleared up. I feel serene, content. I know that everything is going to work out all right. I feel a sense of relaxation and a lack of urgency about doing anything. Life, problems, people, pain, so what? A feeling of both exhilaration and peace with the world. I am exceedingly happy. I want to laugh and smile for no reason. I feel my state of exaltation, waxing and waning." L.B., a volunteer, wrote: "I was very frightened with my memories. It was a great emotional shock for me. . . . As a result of LSD, I like myself better. I'm doing more for myself in many little ways." Another volunteer gained significant personality insights into himself." He wrote: "I chose forever to give up ideas of power over myself and others in exchange for the feeling of well-being and humor." Another volunteer participated in the birth and delivery of a small baby—herself. She went back to her first breath and each new gasp of air was a startlingly joyous experience.

The last of Ludwig's characteristics, also apparent among Janiger's Q-sorts and volunteers reports, is that of hypersuggestibility. Chapter 7 details this phenomenon, but volunteers' reports are full of the need to follow the suggestions of someone, although no one may necessarily have been present to direct the experience: "Others seem to be controlling my thoughts. I feel that they are trying to put something over on me. I was angry because I was so suggestive to whatever I was told to do. I have become very susceptible to suggestion. My mind sometimes becomes a complete blank with no thoughts at all in it. I feel that the music was controlling everything, including me. I have an almost hypnotic compulsion to execute suggestions. It was easier to agree than to resist. I felt very amenable to all suggestions or requests." A woman volunteer wrote that LSD stripped her to the naked core of her own particular actions and reactions, a stripping to the bone of her basic thinking and behavior patterns that with proper conditioning might establish new reactions and insight. She compared her experience to hypnosis, which she had recently undergone, reflecting that both made her feel that she was observing herself apart from her being. She wrote: "I believe both hypnotism and LSD work on the subconscious through suggestion and conditioning, if a person were to be brought to a hypnotic state and then given LSD, the power of the drug would really tell."

Janiger's constants also included a number of effects that were not part of a general global response to altered states of consciousness. Mostly, they included negative responses that were due to the effect of the LSD and the volunteers' lack of prior knowledge or expectation. While most people typically seek out altered states of consciousness for socially-approved goals and with the expectation of specific benefits, in Janiger's study the expectations were minimal and people were caught unaware when the experience became exceedingly intense. Thus many of Janiger's categories of effects included negative experiences of hallucinations, anxiety and fear, strong physical alterations including cramps, paralysis, and agony, paranoid feelings, depression, guilt, and irritation, somatic discomfort, strange body feelings, inhibitions, unreality, strangeness, and disappointment. Some of the volunteers' words illustrate these negative responses. We quote liberally from the reports. "I began to feel weak behind my knees. My hand looked like a relief map of hills and deep cut gorges. I went to the toilet, and as I urinated it seemed the water would never stop. Huge quantities of fluid left my body and I was shrinking and drying up. I had many somatic feelings. My left side felt chained and in a sticky gray mire." Another volunteer wrote: "There were two of me, side by side, as in a blur. I was disappointed because I felt I was only one thing all day—a little girl and that none of my other feelings came out." A film coordinator wrote that she could barely manage to sit up without becoming ill. Another man had fits of cold and depression, feelings of aloneness and a lack of protection and love. He wrote: "I imagined myself in the place of those less fortunate who are behind hospital walls for mental illness. They were laughing at me behind my back or up their sleeves." Another woman wrote: "I was briefly exploding volcanoes and with each eruption my body violently shuddered and shook. I heard the forlorn beseechingly lonely sobbing of all childhood, restricted inner sobbing held within by an agony of repression. Then came the deep cries of weeping adults, men and women and moaning and groaning." Another wrote: "It was a pure horror experience. Persistent vibrating noise like a jackhammer beating away in my brain incessantly for a long time. My equilibrium was very poor."

Ludwig argues for understanding both the benefits and dangers of the altered state of consciousness. The reader, by now, has noted the overwhelming nature of negative experiences reported by volunteers, even in the larger context of enlightening artistic, spiritual, or therapeutic breakthroughs. While at first blush this appears to be paradoxical, the phenomenon of abreacton, or catharsis, is clearly occurring here. This concept describes the release of emotions as the result of recalling or reliving a traumatic, repressed experience with which they are associated. Catharsis is the purifying of the emotions or the relieving of emotional tension, which is often facilitated by art. In his *Poetics,* Aristotle articulated his expectation that drama should be accompanied by a cathartic experience for the viewer. From a psychiatric perspective, abreaction alleviates people's fears, problems, and complexes by bringing them to consciousness or giving them expression. The mundane concept of "no pain, no gain" applies here. While the LSD constants include many negative-sounding categories, in their narratives most volunteers jump from these commentaries to accounts of meaningful personal experiences such as seeing the crucifixion of Christ or being able to break out from under deep inhibitions that limit their life choices.

This book does not attempt to apply any kind of independent standard of measurement to evaluate Janiger's data. Rather, like many western psychocultural studies based on self-reported information, we focus on the perceptions of individuals who have these experiences and the meanings that the experiences have for them. From this we then try to determine their implications for further study. The data raise far more questions than they answer. Are the effects of LSD simply transitory and illusory? Are people self-deceiving about their experiences? Is the art produced during or after LSD superior? And so on. For our purposes as we try to understand Janiger's data, we can certainly see that the LSD experience can create a way to open avenues to new realms of experience, new knowledge, artistic inspiration, and religious, revelatory, or prophetic insights. The heightened aesthetic sensibilities of the psychedelic experience clearly broaden the individual's subjective sensitivities. In the great majority of reports we see instances in which moral values were affirmed, emotional conflicts were resolved, and participants appear to have been better able to cope with human predicaments. In the next chapter, a review of follow-up studies conducted some forty years later will permit us to see the lasting effects, if any, of these fateful days in Wilton Place, Los Angeles.

THE VOLUNTEERS SPEAK FOR THEMSELVES

The following material consists of phrases taken directly from the Q-sort cards during the early stages of the experiment. Like the excerpts above, each section may include statements from several volunteers. Whenever possible the comments are presented in the first person, which is the way that the volunteers reacted to the Q-sort—in terms of their own subjective experiences.

Real, Visual, and Auditory Hallucinations

There is a strange taste in my mouth. I hear things I know are not real. I can make an object turn into something else just by wanting it to. There are very vivid scenes, which seem very real at the time. I see and hear things happening, which couldn't be happening, and yet they seem very real. The things I see out of nowhere seem like they're really there. I see faces of little animals coming out of the walls. I can picture anything I wish. I see people or animals in motion, who aren't really there. I have the illusion of smelling something which isn't there. I can smell something very strongly. At times, I have the sensation of something or someone touching me. I heard wonderful music playing, only there wasn't any. I keep hearing music that isn't being played. People, some of whom I'd known in the past, others right out of thin air appear. I hear voices. Ants are walking where there weren't any ants. I see horrible looking faces. Sometimes I could hear the sound of my voice and other times I wasn't sure whether all these things running through my mind were said out loud or not. I lived through the sensation of being many different types of people, all horrible. Hallucinations of almost a cosmic nature. Waves of hallucinations of anal, visceral and bloody order. There were things crawling on the walls. The wallpaper seemed to be weeping. All the sounds were far away.

Anxiety and Fear

I am fearful of misplacing things. I have a sense of urgency that I have to do it right now. Certain things are frightening me. It's not very safe to experiment like this. I have some fear that I might become permanently insane. I feel anxious or fearful. I'm afraid that I will tremble uncontrollably when I use my hands but when I try it, I surprise myself by doing so well. I'm afraid to get up and walk but then I surprised myself that I could do it so well without staggering; I don't like letting loose of my hold on sanity this way. I seem to be on the fringes of sheer horror or fearful that something dreadful is about to happen; I have a feeling of wanting to escape. I'm caught in terror, a struggle, an agony, the essence of blackness. Help! Panic. I'm caught. I feel a sense of nameless terror all about me. I fear that I will lose control and scream. I feel apprehensive. I fear that the effects might last. I fear that if I continue to keep my eyes closed, I may sink out of sight. I have never known such a complete and utter state of helplessness. Waves of panic would start to flood through me. I was terrified only it was a terror beyond terror. Everything seemed to fall apart. I was afraid of being absolutely and irrevocably obliterated. I was afraid of being alone. I was frightened merely of crossing the room. There was nothing to hang on to. I seemed to suffer the greatest anxiety and fear in enclosed places. I felt so desperate that I called for help. I had a feeling of falling into some bottomless place which was simply terrifying.

Cramps, Paralysis, and Agony

This is the most agonizing thing I've ever experienced in my life. I feel that I am dying or about to do so. I am in agony. I feel cramps in my stomach. I feel my heart beating harder and faster than usual. There is pressure in my head and behind my eyeballs. I am more aware of my heartbeat than usual. Everything seems too bright, too harsh, or too loud. I feel paralyzed. I can hardly move a muscle. There is pressure in my ears. I have much difficulty in breathing. I feel choked. I can hardly breathe. My joints ache and my muscles feel cramped. My body is being pummeled, squeezed, knotted, or twisted. I feel that the dosage was too high. It takes great effort to move, to stand up or to walk. The whole experiment has been hell to me. I thought I was strangling. I was in an agony of physical pain.

Paranoid Feelings

I am suspicious of the intentions of the people around me. I hear the voices of people who are trying to kill me. I overhear people plotting against me. I feel threatened with bodily harm. I'm really not as smart as I think I am. These doctors think they know it all. I can influence the thinking and actions of people and objects with my thoughts. I know that I am not really being persecuted, even though I seem to feel that way. They are making fun of me. They don't think that what I say is important. I suspect some kind of trick. They're purposely irritating me. I resent what they're doing to me. Others seem to be controlling my thoughts. They don't know how important this is to me. I feel that they are trying to put something over on me. I have the impression that people are talking against me. Other people must know that there is something wrong with me. In a public place I feel I must be making an awful fool of myself. I can hear people scheming against me. I feel suspicious. Other people seem to be talking about me, even when I know they weren't. It seems to me that people became very menacing and frightening to look at. I have a feeling that my appearance has changed. I feel that all that I am expe-

riencing is being suggested to me by the therapist. It seems like everything is being manipulated. People look sinister or threatening. Violence. They're coming after me. I'm frightened. People seemed sinister and threatening. The atmosphere seemed to be charged with a real, but unfocused danger. This is a mental institution and all are watching me. Intonations became significant and loaded with inference, reference, plot. I was angry because I was so suggestive to whatever I was told to do. I would lift the curtain to see if the street was still there. I felt a sense of cunning. I shouted, cursed and demanded attention as well as obedience.

Depression, Guilt, and Irritation

I don't like the way things look. I have thought of suicide. I feel remorseful. Depression would start but I'd just shake it off. A feeling of desolation and sadness. Not anger, no regrets, just desolation. All is grim, tawdry, frightening and unpleasant. I want what I want, right now, when I want it. I feel damned. No relief. I dislike distractions much more than usual. Everything seems futile. I dislike interruptions like people butting in while I'm trying to think. I get furious at people for interfering with me. I just can't tolerate anything which isn't just what I want. I am feeling much anger and irritation. I experienced a great demand for perfection in everything I saw. I was more critical and yet more appreciative. A sense of frustration and anger, or fury. The music helps to blot out distractions. I had a feeling of wanting to explode but not being able to. I feel stupid. I know what it is like to be dead, physically dead. Life seems to have lost its meaning. I feel depressed. Everything feels hopeless. Things having to do with death kept coming to mind. I feel very guilty over things I've done in the past. I misunderstand and build up a case over little things people do. I feel remorse over things gone by. The music was just annoying, not enjoyable, like two programs coming over the radio at the same time. Everything said by others seems inane or pointless. I dislike all this very much. It makes me angry to have people hurry me or tell me what to do. If it got any worse, I don't know if I can stand it. It's getting to be too much. I think I'm feeling the way an insane person must feel. My conscience seems to be bothering me. Why can't those people shut up and stop bothering me. The only thing I objected to was me. I didn't like myself. In the mirror I saw nothing that wasn't ugly. I felt there was something in what they were saying that I was too stupid to understand. I was afloat in the world, utterly desolately alone. There never was such a sense of separateness, isolation. I felt so strange, sick, along and most of all, helpless. I became aware of some awful and ill-defined revelation as if I had come across a great personal truth, as if I were only minutes away from the end of being. I am damned. A darkness settled over my mind and I knew this was death. I alternated between depression and mild euphoria. There was no fear in me, only a sorrow as big as all imaginable space. I wanted to kill. An overpowering rage consumed me. I was filled with a vast explosive impatience. I found myself becoming increasingly annoyed and irritated with intrusions upon my world of enchantment. People, traffic, noise were repugnant. Other people's movement became increasingly oppressive to me. I had to shield my eyes as they moved about. I cannot stand any intervention or distraction by anybody. The pressure of any will, anyone making a suggestion or asking a questions presses almost physically on my naked brain.

Somatic Discomfort

I am trembling inside. I am shaking very badly. I feel shaky inside but it doesn't show. I am having chills. I feel felt upset and nervous. A sense of nervous tension is never at anytime absent during the experience. Impossible to relax. I want to rest and get really comfortable, but I can't. I feel a sense of restlessness like I've never known. I feel the need to stretch my muscles or have to get moving, walking, dancing, or going for a drive. I feel a sense of nervous tenseness inside. I'm feeling tense. The experience was, on the whole, very unpleasant for me. I was worrying much about something during the 24 hours before the experience began. I had only a little sleep the night before the experience began. I felt a different kind of headache than I've ever had before. My head aches like in a usual sort of way. Strange feelings in the front of my head or the base of my skull but not quite a headache. I felt struggle, agony, clutching, gasping, clawing, a coldness in my chest, a wringing of hands. The experience was mainly uncomfortable and painful for me. There was little or no enjoyment that wasn't mixed with pain. Food was interesting only to look at. I was relieved to come out of the most intense phases of the experience. I had to urinate more often than usual. I had to vomit. Various parts of me are jerking. My mouth is very dry. I have funny feelings on my skin. I am sweating. I feel weak. I feel so nauseated that I can throw up. My stomach feels a little upset. I get dizzy. I am getting restless. My left hand is real numb. I was terribly restless and unable to stop my pacing. I was ready to moan out loud with the physical distress I was experiencing. Hunger was like a gnawing hole in my stomach.

Strange Body Feelings

My voice sounds different. One half of my body felt differently from the other half. It's as if part of me were split off and independent of the rest. Parts of my body don't seem to belong to me. The shape of my body doesn't seem normal. I am aware of things about parts of me that I wasn't aware of before. The left side of my body is reacting more strangely than the right side. It seems as if my body is about to break apart in pieces. I have no desire for food at all. Part of me feels numb. My arms and legs feel like lead. I have a burning sensation in parts of my body. I feel tingling chills at certain sensitive or private points. My body is annoying me. Funny changes, as if my teeth were falling out or there was a wafer stuck to the roof of my mouth. My bodily motions feel different, somewhat hard to coordinate. I can't help crying. I feel a warm glow all over. My hands and feet feel light. I feel unsteady. I seem to have no body at all. My body seems to be doing strange things all on its own, changing in size, growing younger or older. My hands and feet feel peculiar. I feel like I'm floating in space. My body feels light. I am soaring. I am much more aware of my own motion than usual. I feel as if I am melting, disintegrating, turning into a liquid. I suddenly find myself about 15 feet tall. I felt like a pygmy. I felt I was trembling and yet I wasn't when I studied my hands. My body felt gross and an encumbrance to my senses. I had very little consciousness of my body. It feels light, remote and insubstantial. Parts of my body felt as if they were flowing away. The impression I received was of my body being in another dimension.

Dreamy and Hypnogogic

My eyesight seems blurred. I have trouble focusing my eyes. To speak, or act upon anything has become a real problem for me. I just want to lie down and rest. Matters of sex keep coming to mind. I have become very susceptible to suggestion. My mind sometimes becomes a complete blank with no thoughts at all in it. I feel that the music was controlling everything, including me. It's almost like dreaming. I can hear things much more loudly. Music affects my mood much more intensely than usual. I am transported by music; what I see, think, feel, are all taken over by its power. What I'm thinking about gets shattered by noises, which seem too loud. I hear voices or noises which aren't there, sort of like when dreaming. Reality, harsh reality—it gets in the way. Felt as if I'd been to so many places and I know I've been here all the time. It needs an effort to keep attentive to the real scene and not drift into the vision world. An almost hypnotic compulsion to execute suggestions. It was easier to agree than to resist. I felt very amenable to all suggestions or requests.

Internal—Visual Images and Synesthesia

Sometimes with my eyes closed I see spectacular performances and dancing. Exotic objects or scenes from foreign lands pass before my eyes. Sounds seem to affect what I see. I see music; the textures of rhythms and the colors of melodies float before my eyes. My visual images alter or change whenever I hear a sound or noise. I feel like I am seeing colors for the first time. Brilliant gems in marvelous settings, velvets and lace and jewelry appear. With eyes closed, there are harmonious beautiful colors and textures, gorgeous gems in wonderful settings. Sight, feeling, motion, color, texture, thinking, sound—all are one. The music is fantastic and with it, fantastic imagery. Many different kinds of visual images, often suggested by the mood of the music. The interaction and interplay between sight, music, and physical feeling is most remarkable. I seem to be seeing things after I stopped looking at them, a sort of after-image. I know where I am and what's going on and that these strange changes I'm seeing are not really taking place. Even when things looked different, I knew they had not actually changed. The walls flap in the breeze like tapestries. They run like melted wax. The floor flows like a river. The folds and textures of cloth become rich and wonderful to look at. Lights seem to change gradually. The air seems to have become textured, colored or with structure, particularly near the corners of objects. I have been able to imagine and see beautiful vivid landscapes or architecture. With my eyes closed, I see multi-colored moving designs. I see flashing lights or colors when I close my eyes. With my eyes closed, I notice bright clear pictures of objects or symbols. With my eyes closed, I see a procession of multi-hued metamorphosing (ever changing) fantastic images. With my eyes closed, I see a complex pattern like a church window or arches and passageways in a temple. When I close my eyes, the effects of the drug seem to become more intense. When I close my eyes and concentrate, I can sometimes see dancing girls or other spectacular performances. Colors around me seemed brighter. When I closed my eyes, *there were blinding flashes of light. When you close your eyes, you just lose yourself in an orgy of sensation. You see architectural shapes mixed to natural ones. Losing yourself in feeling. The visions that appeared before my closed eyes filled me with horror. Fantastic forms, dripping, changing, everything in slow motion, twisting, spiraling shapes turning into other shapes. The music translated into a remarkable succession of pictures in my imagination.*

Perceptual Distortions

Vibrations are visible to me. I smell something that I know is not really there. Seeing double without actually seeing double, like seeing objects through shimmering air. Difficulty in picking up objects as if they were stuck in wax or glue. Objects acted like they were stuck in wax when I try to lift them. Objects seemed to move more fluidly when they move. Things seem magnified, coarse, unpleasantly spotted and larger than usual. Other people's faces seem to have become changing masks. Looking in the mirror, the recognition of the expressions in my face seem to be out of phase with the visual images. My own face in the mirror looks fantastically different. Suddenly it will become fluid and then change into several faces at once. In the mirror, my face is like putty, soft and pliable, changing horribly. Things seemed to be moving by themselves, a life of their own. Things don't seem to be the right shape any more. Peoples' faces are grotesque. I seem to be more keenly aware of things like wind and motion, and the senses of touch or weight or posture. My hearing seem sharper than usual. I seem to have developed X-ray vision. Walls or other objects seem to be breathing. Things seem to move away or come closer. The walls do not meet at right angles anymore. There is a wavering, fluid motion to solid objects. Things seem to change in shape or proportion. Objects seem to be superimposed on themselves in a strange, fluid fashion. Flat surfaces have parts sticking out several inches in front of them. Depth perceptions altered with flat surfaces seeming to have some portions brought forward and other parts set back. My sense of depth perception seems to have changed. I've lost the ability to judge distances. Details stand out boldly like cracks and imperfection.

The subtle colors in things stand out. Pictures seem to have a third dimension that I've never noticed before. Ordinarily flat pictures take on a striking three-dimensional quality. Objects seemed to glow around the edges. Colors and objects seem to glow with their own source of light. What I see flows over into the next thing that I see. The thing I look at changes before my very eyes. I have to struggle to keep things in control. Seeing things in a new way. The room is at an angle like a tipped plane.

Inhibitions

It's amazing what it's like to be really oneself. I felt I didn't want to loosen up and let things happen. I can't seem to let myself go as much as I'd like to. I'm afraid I will tell secret things. I have a sense of my own individuality—as if no one could help me but me and this is very satisfying. It seems easier to express things I ordinarily keep hidden. I feel like talking about things I'd never talked about before. I like to talk about what I am seeing or feeling. I feel terrible about what I'm thinking. I feel more myself than I ever was before. I feel worried that my thoughts will show. I'm afraid that someone will see the things in me that I don't want seen. A feeling of being psychologically undressed, even in the dark. There are things I want to say but fear stops me. Wanting to express certain things but feeling I shouldn't. The effect of LSD seemed to remove my reluctance to discuss or even think about certain phases of my experiences. I began to experience a mounting excitement, which reminded me of childish emotions. I described my state as one of "psychic incontinence." Giggling grotesquely while inside of me were locked up sane and reasonable thoughts. I would not have ordinarily blurted out my feelings so easily.

Confusion and Mind Flooded

I feel confused but can't explain in what way. I have trouble understanding what is being said. My mind doesn't seem to make sense out of what my body is doing but my body seems to function all right by itself. Fighting hard to concentrate and not being able to do so. My thoughts are all jumbled up. I feel I have some control over the experience that I can pull out of it to some extent if I need to. It is very difficult for me to try to concentrate on anything without increasing my feeling of sickness such as nausea, headaches, backaches, etc. Everything seems sort of confused. No control over my mind anymore. I was relieved to get back to the place where I could organize my thinking. I keep desperately trying to concentrate, trying to clear the confusion. This isn't so painful, but why do I get lost? I have become aware of things going on in my mind that are quite beyond description. There are levels of my thought not reached by what I say. I can see my thinking process. It is possible to observe my thoughts clearly and separately, even when there appears to be many of them at once. My thoughts are all connected, each flowing into the other. Pulling one thought out of a stream of ideas and tried to analyze it before the next thought distracted one. My mind is flooded with thoughts, I can't seem to think straight. I felt overwhelmed by what was happening to me and incompetent to explain my feelings. Let me return to reality for just one moment so that I could catch my breath and get oriented again. It was very difficult to finish a sentence or thought. Words, ideas, concepts, rushed in and out of my consciousness. I lose my capacity to synthesize. I was confused as to my precise location. I was fairly lucid, but wasn't able to think back. I was slow to connect sounds or sights with what they actually meant. There are moments which I do not remember, when I was in and out of it. One of the weirdest sensations was the in and out quality of my consciousness; of being thrust back and forth from blankness to awareness. You feel as though you're in the middle of a whirlpool, a little bit. You know you can let yourself go or not. I could fight it but why bother.

Attention, Communication, Short-term Memory

I feel more talkative than usual. I have trouble remembering what I was doing a few seconds ago. I keep forgetting where I am and how I spent the last few minutes getting there. I seem to be easily distracted. I find that my interest lags when I try to complete something. Disturbing to my ability to think things out and to communicate my ideas. My interest in things is sharpened and yet I can't keep my attention on any one thing for very long. My mind jumps from one thing to another. I keep thinking a senseless thing over and over. The words you hear yourself saying sometimes sound completely idiotic. I blanked out completely for a while. The experience seemed a little fuzzy, and I'm not sure I remember all of it clearly. The experience now seems pretty hazy to me with blank spots as to what happened at times. My memory seems poorer than usual. I find myself saying things I don't believe. There are long pauses between my words in which I am attending to many other and different thoughts, which have nothing to do with what I am saying. I have difficulty talking but it doesn't seem to matter. I hear my mouth saying words that didn't seem to make much sense to me. For a while, I wasn't conscious of being in the room there at all. I change my mind in the middle of a sentence. Something I was going to say sounds rather void of meaning after I think it over. I feel that my speech is slurred. Words seem to be stumbling blocks. I start a sentence and halfway through, I forget what I was trying to *say; I forget the first part of a sentence before I finish it but sometimes it will come back after a while if I wait for it. Ideas are forming so fast that I can't state them all. I keep forgetting what I was talking about in the middle of a sentence. I kept forgetting what I was thinking about right in the middle of a sentence. I find difficulty in remembering certain words that I want to use. I have to talk around them to describe their meaning. It is impossible to have a thought and then express it before you forget what it is. Each moment seemed completely new with no past members to explain it. Ideas interrupt each other. Speech is difficult, not because ideas are coming so fast, but because of a blankness, a forgetting, of being unable to hang onto an idea. I can't remember what I started to think. I sometimes lose interest in what I've started saying, so that a sentence gets left unfinished. I was easily distracted by details. I talked at length and much of it seemed like babbling to me but I didn't care.*

Unreality, Newness, Strangeness

Everything seemed brittle, thin and unreal. Other people seem to lack substance. No longer the security of the ordinarily accepted foundations of logical thinking, no stable reference points to cling to, no absolutes, no fixed basis for the usual rules of living. A feeling of not really being in the room. At the same time, everything seemed so real, so vivid. Much of the experience seemed artificial, the visual experiences were too gaudy, too lacking in substance. No longer in this world. A lot of what happened during the experience seems unreal. I feel that in normal everyday living there is much that is being withheld from us, that there actually is another dimension that we can't ordinarily get into. No purpose to the nature of things as they really are. The foundations are washed out from under everything that seemed fundamental or important. I find myself in another dimension, in a new, entirely different dimension. What is meaning? verbal? sensory? physiological or what? The touch of someone's hand helps to bring me back when I'm far out. Just like sunrise, in a strange town after an all-night drive in a car, everything so sharp and clear and yet inside, a strange nervousness. Everything seems unreal. Everything has a sense of awesomeness, amazement and wonder about it. I feel I am in contact with the unknown. My thinking seems to have become tied to or equal to one or another of my senses, like sight, smell or posture. A growing sense of unreality of my surroundings. the subjective feeling of living in the sense of feeling, sensing, is perhaps the only reality.

The possibility struck me that what I was experiencing was not real. I suddenly developed a great fear of becoming lost in unreality. Reality had become too fluid for me. There were levels to reality. When I returned to what seemed to be reality, I came from a great distance. The feeling of being submerged under water. I'm under glass where people can look at you. I feel as though I were surrounded by a membrane. All stimuli coming from all directions with equal intensity and flattening out against the membrane. The outside world seemed muffled. The world looks agreeably disassociated from me. I was aware of a sense of strangeness in relation to my surroundings, a disorientation which persisted throughout the experience. I was seeing again with infantile newness. This is my first day on earth.

Recall and Reliving

Funny how you can remember things so clearly. Memories of childhood return to me. Just like a little 5 or 10 year old kid, not knowing what to do, or who to turn to for help, and yet I was an adult, looking on and watching myself. I am reminded of a dream that I can never remember. I keep thinking of many of my problems. Things I am remembering throw a new light on some of my problems. I can quickly scan over and re-live many parts of my life. I have a very vivid recall of scenes and emotions from days gone by. I actually seem to return to certain moments in childhood and experience myself there. I sense things about myself which I don't like. I lived through one or two experiences in my life. A distinct quality of "deja vu." The feeling which I must have felt as an infant, or perhaps even before that. I began to feel like a little girl. I was astounded by the fund of knowledge available to me as I made references to literature, art, and mythology that I had not thought of for years.

Alertness

Compared to this, the usual ways of seeing things are flat and uninteresting. Small details seem to stand out more than usual. I have the feeling of being on the verge of an important revelation but not quite able to express it. I see everything more intensely. There is a greater desire to be exact in my descriptions. I feel extremely alert. Certain objects suddenly stand out. My mind seems greatly improved. A feeling of excitement and anticipation, like when something very important is about to happen. I can remember very clearly everything that happened to me during the experience. There's a feeling of seeing things more clearly. I could see miles away even noticing the detailed markings of birds in flight from afar. I could figure out anything and felt that nothing was complicated and I understood everything so clearly. I was aware of myself to the roots of my hair. My thinking seemed much clearer.

Importance, Purpose, Meaning, Real

I suddenly realized that I've been unnecessarily and needlessly condemning myself. I feel more creative than usual. Things that I thought were important don't seem that way now. I've become more aware of unimportant things. I feel that I now know the real meaning of things. I can understand some things far better than before. Not the usual verbal conscious changes in attitudes and feelings, but something much deeper. I know now that many things in life are shallow. I can see that there's a lot of wasted effort in my life. I know better what to do in the future. There seems to be a shift in values from material to non-material. It seems easier than usual to decide what I want. I see the falseness of the various roles that I have been playing, roles, which I once thought were really "myself." I see now that life is, on the whole, wrongly understood and wrongly used, to ends which are really quite futile. The most important thing right now to the person is describing what I'm experiencing. The most important things in the world right now are my thoughts. I feel that everything I'm saying is very important. Everything seems to have a symbolic meaning in it. Ordinarily meaningless gestures now seem important. To speak or act, I become undecided between the futility of doing so and the lack of need and the need. It doesn't seem to matter and yet it does matter, much more so than before. I don't seem to care about things that should be important. A sense of things being tremendously important and completely futile at the same time. Only now do I really see the point of existence. Everything somehow seems more real. Objects seem more real. Significance's become more apparent. I know more now what is real. A passionate desire for something, but I don't know what. This experience is showing me an aspect of reality I've never seen before. I seem to be seeing myself as I am. It seems unusually fitting to observe the usual customs and rituals of everyday living.

Appreciation, Depersonalization, and Natural vs. Artificial

Things of a complex surface texture, like a lawn or gravel, seem much more interesting than things of simple textures like metal or plastic. Natural objects were much more exciting than artificial ones, a single leaf—wonderful. The rough ceiling, gravel, carpets became structured in intricate elaborate patterns but they seemed somehow more in my mind than real. Natural things seem so different from artificial objects. They seem somehow better organized. The distinction between natural and artificial things was much more pronounced. The natural things had a richness, a meaningfulness which the others didn't. Inside of me and outside of me: the subject-object distinction is no longer clear. I'm inside of me, and outside of me at the same time. The distinction between self and non-self becomes less evident. I can put myself consciously into the place of the artist who was painting the picture. I feel I am sharing the meaning of music or art with the artist himself who wrote, played, or painted it. My self-boundaries seemed to expand until other people or objects were included within myself. I feel I can take on the nature or personality of some object or animal or person and yet remain myself. I seem to be able to watch myself like an observer. My conscious mind seemed to be watching my subconscious. I seem to be outside myself looking in. I feel I have several identities, only one of which is the usual "me." I believe that in the future, the appreciation of beauty will play a greater part in my life. My aesthetic appreciation seems improved. I can understand the structure and meaning of music as never before. LSD opened up a whole new world of appreciation and beauty. There's a new tonal sharpness to music. The music is compellingly beautiful. I was able to hear several parts of the orchestra individually at the same time, and almost analyze the individual notes. I can be looking at some object and pretty soon I am not sure which is the object and which is me. My voice has a detached quality. Funny things happen to your sense of ego. A sort of double personality permits me to be and at the same time to observe from the outside.

Mystical

Words are inadequate. None of these cards really adequately describe what I was experiencing. The experience was concrete rather than verbal and indescribable. Everything is interrelated with everything else in a way which ordinarily wouldn't seem possible. There is no such thing as cause and effect. Everything just happens of its own accord. Everything seems explained. Plants and flowers have an extraordinary inner meaningfulness to them. I can see all the mysteries of the universe in a single leaf. Black and white, good and bad, etc. are now mysteriously connected with each other. Opposites seem to be related in a strange paradoxical ways. Things I look at have a new wonderful inexpressible meaningfulness. Everything is exactly right, just as it is. All things are beyond judgment and comparison, beyond morale and simply exist by right of their own perception. Everything has its rightful place in life, even though we call some things good and others bad. Love, the existence of some over-all Creator or Order to the Universe, an Unknown source, something like this seems more possible now. There seems to be a pattern inherent in everything. The whole universe is one and there is no separation into individuals. I feel closer to God. I seem to be in tune with nature. Everything seems to harmonize. The possibility of wonderful new intellectual and philosophical relationships present themselves. I feel a sense of wonder, joy and wholly peaceful inevitableness to the world. The patterns and colors I find in objects and walls fill me with an amazed wonder and acceptance by their mere existence. To be alone with nature is wonderful. I feel like praying. A sense of deeper understanding of love and hate, good and bad. This was the true meaning of eternity. I was conscious of some large pulsation of the earth and its ageless elements and I felt myself to be part of them. A feeling of oneness with nature. It was like being at the bowels of the earth at the beginning of time. I felt an enormous awe, almost religious. An acute awareness of pattern in everything surrounding me—all patterns within patterns. I felt on the verge of some Great Understanding, that with a little straining, I could have the explanation for everything. I studied the plant lovingly and felt that in some way it represented all of life. I am all the tears and sorrow in the world. I was composed of all the love and sympathy in the world. I feel a sudden inexplicable tenderness. All one's experiences are like messages received from an unseen power. I was overcome by a great feeling of love, but I didn't know for whom the beauty and truth of one object would have been enough to keep me fascinated and awed for a lifetime, I deeply resented the intrusion of civilization upon nature. I was suspended in eternity, convinced that this was the same place souls go.

Relaxation and Quiet

A certain inner quietness, instead of all the mixed-up jumble of everyday life. I feel more relaxed than usual. The physical symptoms I had when I came in seemed to have cleared up. I feel a general philosophical sadness over things which cannot be altered. I feel serene, content, knowing. I have no desire to move. Now, I know that everything is going to work out all right.

All of the petty incidents of everyday life, which tended to irritate me, seem relieved, seem not to bother me any more. There is a deeper awareness of the general fitness of things, of the acceptance of things as they are. Such complete relaxation, so much enjoyment. A number of things that had been bothering me suddenly seemed solved. I feel much calmer than usual. I seem to be much quieter than usual. I now have a new kind of philosophic attitude. I feel a sense of relaxation and a lack of urgency about doing anything. Life, problems, people, pain, so what? No bother, it all makes no difference. I just want to sit and keep looking at an object for hours on end. I just like to sit and meditate with my eyes closed, seeing what happens and not stopping it. I was content to passively receive large scale and diffused impressions, I wanted to avoid anything that would intrude on the privacy and peace. I don't want to open my eyes. I was in my own private world, glowingly warm, wonderfully silent and I wanted to stay there forever. A feeling of both exhilaration and peace with the world. I preferred most of all to contemplate and to look at the wondrous visions that crossed my lowered eyelids. A relaxed lack of concern with the world.

Euphoria and Laughter

This is probably better than I've ever felt before so far as a sense of well-being is concerned. My face seems to form itself into a grin, quite without my will or control. I'm hungry. I'm unable to control my feelings. I can't control this laughter. I feel pleasant and comfortable. The experience was the greatest thing that ever happened to me. It was very enjoyable. I would like to try this again some time. I feel that the experience was beneficial and worthwhile. I feel exhilarated. I am exceedingly happy and having a wonderful time. There is a human or a jolly atmosphere in our group. I feel pleasantly amused. Everything seems delightfully funny. I would like the state to go on and on for days and days. This is ecstasy. I feel that this was all made just for me. I was laughing as if I would never stop. Things struck me as funny which wouldn't ordinarily seem funny. I became amused at my own thought processes. The experience had both pleasant and unpleasant aspects to it. It was a marvelous experience. I feel more playful than usual. I'm in a very happy mood today. I'm having many different moods. I have violent mood swings from feeling wonderful to feeling terrible. Release, freedom, escape. Would have loved to have gone on like that for hours. I did not want it to completely wear off. I want to laugh and smile for no reason. I wanted to laugh uproariously. This is a big joke on the world. Walking was enormously enjoyable. I am amused, charmed. Extraordinarily happy and contented. I felt lifted up into an area of great contentment and happiness. I felt my state of exaltation waxing and waning. I feel happy but more than happy, silly. It is half unpleasant, half terribly pleasant. When I laughed I cried, and when I cried, I laughed. Even laughed and cried at the same time. I think I'm going to laugh and it comes out a tear.

Comparisons with Drinking Behavior

Oh, for a drink of whisky to get rid of this feeling. This is the only time I ever had such a craving for alcohol while sober. I feel very drunk. This is almost like the DTs. I went through exactly the same stages as when I'm drinking. The experience almost drove me to drink. Brings back the DTs, fears and horrors. I ache in exactly the same places I do during certain other types of experiences. At times, I felt like I wanted a drink. Just like a hangover. I walk in feeling inferior and after a couple of hours, I feel like I own the place. I felt just like I was drinking. I've tried to get this same feeling from drinking but never quite made it. The experience left me feeling like I wanted a drink. An exact duplicate of my first few years of drinking history. I feel more confident of my ability to stop drinking. I've lost my illusions about drinking now. I've not fooled anyone, only myself. I feel exactly like I've had a couple of drinks or so, just sort of high. Just like cracking up after drinking.

Disappointed or No Reaction

No grand visions or insights at all. I feel the dosage was too low. I was disappointed by the experience. I wonder why it doesn't have any effect on me. Expecting something to happen, but it didn't. I'm distinctly annoyed because I seem to be getting no reaction. What's the matter with me, nothing's happening. The experience didn't live up to my expectations. Nothing happened. At no time did I have a real serene feeling of well-being. The experience was nothing unusual at all. At no time did I feel terribly depressed or terribly frightened or terribly anything. My hopes and expectations were not fulfilled. I'm experiencing nothing unusual at all; in fact, I am beginning to become bored. As indescribable as the experience had been, I felt as if I had failed its challenge. This is all a little self-conscious. It is neither better nor worse than myself before. Fear that I was not getting enough out of it, *that I might not be cured, even now. Wondering that maybe the drug really didn't affect me.*

Interpersonal Relations

I felt very much part of the group, no sense of sitting off to one side. I enjoy observing the other people present. People are there but I would ignore them. I want to withdraw away from them. A party-like atmosphere. I feel very detached and distant from the people around me. I feel a sense of warmth toward the people around me. I feel absolutely alone. I don't want to be left alone. Acts, done out of consideration for someone else's happiness, seem somehow more numerous now. I can see to the roots of other peoples' personalities and understand what basically motivates them. I feel at one with people around me. I find it enjoyable when certain people are with me. I have become very conscious of subtle interpersonal relationships. The touch of someone's hand is comforting. I feel that the people here understand me. Having a friend near would have been important. Much less resentment than usual. No barriers at all between the people in the experience but a sense of distance from those on the outside. It seems to strengthen emotional bonds of affection. I felt as if I stood out, as if people were staring at me. I feel more tolerant of people. They don't seem to irritate me at all anymore. Other people seem to be in a different world, or different dimension than I am in. I dislike people butting in on me when I'm trying to think. I feel compelled to advise or help other people. People look more attractive to me than usually. I feel closer to people. I'd just like to go off by myself and be alone. I feel different from everybody else. I feel I want to study the various people about me. I don't want people near to me, I don't want them imposing their conversation and ideas on me. I feel more tolerant than usual. I feel like wanting to do things for people. People seem to be arranging themselves into artistic colorful contexts and groupings within the room. I felt no strong attachment to anybody. I felt no compulsion to talk with a particular person. I felt very friendly and enjoyed the company. I loved the world and everybody and myself. An intense yearning for love, protection and acceptance. I seemed to be imbued with an overpowering sense of love for all things. I felt great amounts of warmth, tenderness, and perhaps even love. I felt bombarded with sensations of love. I just sat around and watched everyone.

Experiencing Time

Everything comes in waves, pulsations, vibrations. The effects seem to come and go. I seem to be experiencing things in more than three dimensions. Rhythms and tempos seem to be all right, even when my sense of time has been very much altered. I feel that I know what will happen before it does, like being a jump ahead of time. Now seems forever. All this seems to have happened to me before. Time seems unimportant I can change past events. Past, present and future are all together now. The clock says an hour's gone by but it just seems like a few seconds. My sense of time seems changed, warped, turned inside out or something.

Time isn't. Time perception very much slowed, falling objects seem to drift slowly to the floor. Time seems to have become one of the dimensions of space. Time seems to be so fleeting. An odd, remote timelessness. Time seemed to have come to a complete standstill. Three long years into one horrible few minutes. A disorientation in time and all events seemed to take longer to perform than in reality. Every minute seemed hours and time was dragging.

Orgiastic

The lower half of my body was engulfed in a warm tide of sensation. A distinct feeling of a kind of radiation or pulsation to the limbs, stomach and genital area, of a sensual but not overtly sexual nature. I began to experience very strong feelings of sensuality in and around my belly and the inside of my thighs. My body had begun to experience first tingling then thrills. Then I was engulfed in an uncontrollable sensation, which can only be described as an ejaculation. In reality, I experienced neither erection nor emission. Melting in a fragile state of orgasm that seemed to go on and on, though I knew it was only seconds. I had been experiencing a constant state of what can be described as orgasm, though not in the usual sense. I was wracked with this ecstatic physical feeling. The feelings of sensuality intensified and became rapture of a kind that is almost beyond description. I was in rapture there for a while. The ecstatic physical feeling of surrender became almost overpowering. Pleasurable and somewhat ecstatic as though a gradual loosening of certain sensual and deeper bonds within my body had taken place. These sensual forces of surrender, which I hoped would soon turn me into jelly and splay me out over the countryside in an orgy of pleasure and surrender feast of the senses. The feelings were extremely pleasurable but unlike the usual sexual excitement, I didn't feel the need for gratification. The lack of orgasm does not at all imply any feeling of frustration. I had sexual feelings, which were diffused, undirected and produced a sensation of well-being. The sensual sensations were one-dimensional in that they remained at the same intensity for the whole day. Much more sexual pleasure due to total human consciousness than ecstasy due to sexual experience.

Insightful/Therapeutic

I was aware, as a powerful revelation, of being able to identify my behavior as an old pattern. I seemed to observe a psychotic caricature of my everyday neurotic patterns. It was as if my brain had been placed in my hands, with each hiding place clearly labeled for me to see and know and remember. I realized that was what I was doing in life, going through all the motions without receiving any pleasure, and I would stop this. Provoked a sense of great relief from many years of attenuation of emotion and feeling. It was a wonderful experience and I still enjoy thinking about all the new and wonderful awareness that came from this. I feel as if the boundaries of my consciousness were extended and that I had been given as a gift a new perception of much that is mysterious in human life. LSD provides a revelation of the darkest and most primitive facets and layers of one's being or soul. I am certain that I have never spent as full a day nor extended my senses as far as I did. It was the most creative thing I have ever done and I feel a great satisfaction. The next morning, an uncommon interest in all things surrounding me, a sound sense of self and a general sense of well-being.

Artistic and Creative Insight and Appreciation

I felt I knew exactly what the artist experienced as he painted. As I studied the painting, I felt sure that I had captured the artist's innermost thoughts. My color perception is now exceedingly keen. My color sense became acute. My color and texture perception was very keen. I'm beginning to see what Picasso sees, artists get this kind of a sensation. It's a Van Gogh kind of vision. Every flower, bush and tree standing out in brilliance. I looked at trees for the first time in my life and loved them for the first time. You get the feeling of the exquisite poetry of nature. I still seemed to have a renewed and new appreciation of nature. You develop a kind of intensity of feeling about detail.

The Experience Left Me Feeling . . .

It's not so much the way I feel during it, but the way I feel afterwards that I like. The experience left me with a headache afterwards. The experience left me feeling that it is more important to do something with my life now than before. I feel that If I could have an experience like this every two or three months, I'd never drink again. It left me with a feeling of well-being afterwards. It left me grinning for days. It left me feeling exhausted afterwards. It left me in a state where I couldn't sleep very well afterwards. It left me less impulsive than before. It left me with a more constructive way of thinking than I had before. It left me without a need to always compulsively be doing something all of the time. It left me with a quiet mind. Afterwards, life seemed bleak, futile, hopeless. It left me feeling depressed after it was over. It left me feeling less anxious after it was over, feeling calm and unperturbed after it was over. It left me feeling good, like I haven't felt in months. It left me with a wonderful relief from tension that had been building up. It left me with an increased sense of humor, an ability to laugh and enjoy laughing like I hadn't had for months. It left me with a sense of renewed energy and enthusiasm. It left me tired and worn out. I feel I was helped by it, but nothing earth shaking. It left me feeling happy afterwards. It left me feeling confused about life. It left me feeling not so much in a hurry. It left me feeling shaken. It left me feeling more sure of myself than I was before. It left me with such an untroubled feeling afterwards.

Miscellaneous Comments

My I or self can leave the body and go off to some other part of the room. There is no me. It's like an express train at night with no driver and no brakes. I feel like I am being hurled through the air, as if jet propelled. A repeated hissing sound seems to start at the back of my head and end in an expanding flash of light. The only thing substantial in the world is the touch of someone's hand. Words seem to take on strange new meaning. The whole universe is a tremendous cosmic joke. These drugs certainly have no therapeutic value. They are of no benefit to one's well being. I'd never take it again. There is no good reason for anyone to ever take such drugs. There are too many of these cards. I had a hangover in the morning before I began the experiment. I was well rested when I took LSD. I was in excellent health when the experiment began. I took LSD on an empty stomach. I had been drink-

ing fairly heavily within two days priors to when I took LSD. I do know this, wherever I am, whatever the condition, if this awareness occurs, it will be known as the truth. Total and absolute. Images and symbols have become unnecessary for understanding the real world. Confusion, blacked out. I seem to be capable of mental telepathy. I have a craving for food. I felt they were trying to poison me.

The above accounts represent a cross section of the LSD experiences of the participants and illustrate the LSD constants in considerable detail. Let's turn now to what follow-up studies tell us about the impact LSD made on the lives of Janiger's volunteers.

4

ANALYZING THE
RESULTS OF THE STUDY

AS WE SAW IN CHAPTER 3, many of Janiger's volunteers identified key elements of their LSD experiences in written form on Q-sort cards, and Janiger analyzed the Q-sort data to generate his core constants. It would be fair to say that Janiger's analysis of the Q-sort cards constitutes an informal follow-up study, and the reader is referred to chapter 3 for more details of that process. Additionally, Janiger used questionnaires to tally volunteers' occupations, ages, educational backgrounds, and other demographic data. These questionnaires were sent out to the more than 930 people who participated in the experiment, typically thirty days after their LSD experience. Some seventy percent of the questionnaires were returned, some more promptly than others.

Although much of Janiger's data has never been sifted, an unpublished analysis of almost two hundred returned questionnaires constituted the earliest formal follow-up study and provided notable data on the short-term impact of LSD on Janiger's volunteers' lives. In the late 1990s the Multidisciplinary Association for Psychedelic Research (MAPS) funded a comprehensive follow-up with the goal of identifying both beneficial and detrimental long-term effects of the LSD experience. This chapter surveys both studies. In 1971 Carl Hertel independently analyzed the work of sixty volunteer artists. His results are summarized in the discussion of LSD, art, and creativity in chapter 5. Given the negative press that LSD has had over the years, follow-up studies like the ones discussed in this chapter are absolutely critical in understanding the actual impact of the substance on peoples' lives.

THE INITIAL FOLLOW-UP STUDY

The first follow-up study was conducted more than half a dozen years after Janiger's experiment came to a halt. As summarized in the later comprehensive MAPS study, the initial follow-up analyzed the questionnaire responses of 194 volunteers, who sent their material back to Janiger between 37 and 583 days after their LSD experiences. Even a brief glance at the questionnaire (see appendix I) reveals the breadth of information Janiger sought to gather. Volunteers were asked about any objective changes in their lives since participating in the experiment, such as marriage, divorce, or a new job. They were asked to comment on changes in their relationship to others, such as coworkers, employers, and acquaintances. They were queried regarding increased interest in social reform, political and international affairs, anthropology, moral and ethical issues, and universal concepts. They were asked whether the person closest to them had noted any positive changes or whether they had noted any value changes in their lives, demonstrable in new approaches to issues concerning money, status, and human relationships. Naturally, they were asked whether their LSD experiences were pleasant or unpleasant and whether they would like to try it again. Did they have any religious insights and different understanding of themselves and others? Was there a lasting benefit they obtained from the experience? Finally, the volunteers were asked if LSD should be used by individuals, in general, in order to help them become aware of themselves, to gain new meaning in life, and to help them understand each other better.

The study found that volunteers fell into three groups at the time of their LSD experience: Some volunteers were involved in psychotherapy, and a second group were not in therapy and were drawn from the general population, but excluded physicians and artists, who comprised the last group. The clinical population had a very high rate of positive response to the questions asked of them, much more so than the "average" group. Certainly, the expectations of the clinical group were different because they came to the experiment after recommendation by their psychiatrists or psychologists. The physicians and artists groups also showed a high response rate to positive changes. Additionally, volunteers who had more than four sessions with LSD reported a higher positive response to the effects of LSD. As we will see from the narrative excerpts later in this chapter, however, numerous volunteers did not report a pleasant overall experience, but they nonetheless were glad that they took LSD for the insights they obtained about themselves.

While the clinical volunteers group showed a high rate of positive response overall, they found the LSD experience itself less pleasant than did the "average" group. They also found the experience to have a lasting benefit. The artists, more than others, reported objective changes in their lives. More women than men in the general population group reported positive changes in their relationships to others. Artists reported an increased interest in social reform, political and international affairs, and universal concepts and religion. In contrast, teachers and engineers (a subset of the general population group) reported the least amount of change in this area. Large numbers of artists and men and women in the general population found that positive changes were noted by the person closest to them. Only 12 percent of physicians and psychologists noted this kind of change. Sixty-four percent of the artists queried reported changes in their values. Thirty percent of the physicians and psychologists reported such changes, and 26 percent of men in the general-population sample noticed value changes in themselves.

In all categories queried, the LSD experience was viewed as pleasant overall. This positive response ranged from a low of 56 percent among women volunteers in the general population to a high of 76 percent among teachers and engineers in the general sample. The average woman volunteer appeared ambivalent, and only half agreed that they would like to try LSD again. Among the male volunteers, however, between 71 and 85 percent expressed their desire to take LSD again. When asked whether they now better understood themselves and others, only 32 percent of the physicians and psychologists said yes, while

70 percent of the therapy clients, both men and women, answered positively. When asked how LSD should be used, 43 percent of physicians and psychologists saw it as a way of becoming aware of themselves, 36 percent as a way to gain new meanings to life, and 36 percent as a way to get people to understand each other. In contrast, more than 60 percent of the artists responded positively to each of these questions. Among the psychotherapy group, as many as 84 percent of respondents agreed that the LSD experience made them more aware of themselves.

THE FORTY-YEAR FOLLOW-UP

The MAPS follow-up reported in 1999 presented certain difficulties. After all, just how many people would be alive forty years after the original study concluded, given that the average age of participants at the time of the experiment was early thirties? Not surprisingly, the researchers worked with a fairly small sample. To make the interview process practical, the researchers confined their search for candidates to the Los Angeles area and located forty-eight people. Of these, twelve were referred by Janiger (potentially jeopardizing the sample's capacity to fairly represent the original study population), some were found by a private investigator, and the rest by the interviewer. One person refused to participate in the follow-up, while another was interviewed, but the interview tape came back blank and another tape couldn't be used, leaving a total pool of forty-five respondents plus Janiger, who was also interviewed (Doblin et al. 1999). Naturally, the MAPS researchers had to expect considerable gaps to occur in the perceptual recollection of subjects nearly forty years after the initial study participation, so the follow-up clearly falls into the category of self-reporting without independent verification of forty-year-old memories. In any study, a long lapse in time between the original research endeavor and a follow-up represents a potential threat to the reliability and validity of a research project. The researchers noted these difficulties and were careful to limit their conclusions in view of them.

The MAPS follow-up is important because it provides an unprecedented analysis of LSD's long-term influence on the lives of Janiger's volunteers.

Study Respondents and Research Method

As noted above, the MAPS researchers interviewed Janiger and forty-five of his volunteers—thirty-four men and eleven women, whose average age was 70.3 years when they were contacted for their interviews. A single interviewer conducted and taped all interviews, which ranged between half an hour and more than an hour and were designed to discover how Janiger's volunteers had perceived their LSD experiences and how those experiences had affected their lives in the forty years since. Volunteers were asked what they recalled from their experience, how they viewed their participation in the early research, what effects it had had on their lives, and whether they noted any positive or adverse reactions. Respondents were informed they had the right to halt interviews at will and to remain anonymous in the report. All interview data was analyzed by two researchers, first by the analytic transcriber who identified important data as it emerged during transcription of the tapes, then by a second researcher who used a method specifically designed to "ground" all conclusions in the data.

The researchers found that Janiger's volunteers had learned about his study primarily by word of mouth. In some cases they were in a therapeutic relationship with Dr. Janiger or another psychologist who suggested they take the LSD. Approximately 25 percent of the people interviewed had worked in conjunction with clinicians other than Janiger. In all but one of these cases Janiger administered the LSD at his offices, but the volunteers were accompanied by their own physicians in other settings during the ensuing experiences. As discussed in chapter 3, the inclusion criteria for candidates were wide and the original study pool included an impressive variety of people. All walks of life were similarly represented among the follow-up volunteers.

Results and Conclusions

Of the forty-five people who comprised the final report group, all respondents, with one exception, described their overall LSD experience positively, and approximately one-third of the respondents reported "persisting beneficial changes" that they credited to their participation in Janiger's study. In several cases respondents saw study participation as spiritual or transformative. While interviewees did describe adverse reactions, these were relatively minor and appear to have been short-term.

Nearly all respondents who described their participation in the research felt that it was a positive experience. Many of the volunteers initially described the experience itself in terms of its sensory impact, reporting that LSD enhanced their visual acuity and hearing and that hearing the world became more dramatic than seeing it. One participant, for example, had brought along jazz and classical music and told the interviewer that LSD intensified his hearing acuity. His concentration was increased as well, and the music sounded profoundly beautiful. One man said taking LSD was "the most extraordinary experience of [his] entire life. Nothing before or since has ever come near it." He said it was "like the first time you taste[d] chocolate or the first time you ha[d] an orgasm." He described it as "a genuine peak experience."

Having established the sensory nature of their experiences, many interviewees then offered an emotionally positive interpretation of it. For example, when asked about the effects of LSD on himself, Janiger said in his interview:

> My personal experience is that I've opened the door to some other extension of my mind. Or my sensory equipment or perceptual apparatus. Whatever you want to call it. That gave me access to a kind of world that was vastly enlarged, vastly expanded. And my senses were most acute. My mental capacity of thinking led me to think in terms of breaking away from the familiar, what I called obligatory reality, where I had to be a certain way. It was the first time I clearly saw the influence of society and culture on my development. In other words, I saw how I was literally molded into the person that I was, by being told subtly what to see, what to think, what to feel. And the culture did that subtly. And it started with No and Yes and No and No and No. And I broke out of that completely.

The follow-up showed a consistent pattern of links between the volunteers' emotional, cognitive, and behavioral domains, and the MAPS research team concluded that holistic learning occurred among the volunteers. Many said that their emotional experiences were enhanced. A smaller number described the enhancement of cognitive and behavioral aspects of their experience and changes in their life after their immediate LSD experience.

Perceived long-term benefits occurred in a number of arenas, including changes in worldview, vocations, and interpersonal relationships. One respondent credited his sensory experience with a spiritual awakening. He wrote: "I remember leaving my body and becoming a tree. And I became a tree, went through the roots all through the earth. And I was down in the earth and then I came up through the earth and went into the night sky. And I felt at that point that I'd died and been reborn. But not in a Christian sense! I was raised without religion and I was not spiritual until I took LSD. I've been spiritual ever since." When asked to elaborate, the volunteer said the experience "changed his life forever" and was a "turning point." Another volunteer said that LSD experience eased his fear of death. Another individual who was a psychotherapy patient said that he learned a good deal about himself. He determined that when he was high, he felt himself to be "a much better person than when [he] wasn't" and that his "conventional way of looking at the world and his characterological defenses . . . [had] cut [him] off from much of life's richness." The psychedelic opened him up to these realizations, both aesthetically and emotionally, and stimulated creativity in his thinking.

Several participants reported that their LSD experiences changed the way they conducted their work or the types of work in which they engaged. One volunteer stated that the LSD enhanced his work designing prototypes for the first space vehicles. At the time of his LSD experience, he had been promoted from machinist to researcher— despite having no formal training in this area—because he didn't make mistakes. After participating in Janiger's study, however, he found that he could put his mind right into problems that called for insight and intuition, as nobody really knew anything about them and no one had experience with the materials they were using or developing. The LSD changed the way this participant focused on things and enhanced his problem-solving capabilities. Another man switched his career track from high school physical education to writing metaphysical books and going on lecture tours with Alan Watts. A clergyman changed his focus and subsequently worked for thirty-five years in human consciousness areas.

This same minister found himself temporarily able to lay aside his compulsive cleanliness and anxiety when he came home to a messy house, vastly improving his relationship with his family. He learned what it was like to live as a "non-anxious euphoric being in the world without anxiety or fear of being driven." Content to be, he experienced a new state and was not obsessed with doing, a state that he subsequently "longed for and sought out" for many years.

Such radical transformations, however, were not universal among participants. Almost two-thirds of the study pool reported that they were "not profoundly influenced" by their experiences, which they described simply as "curious and inexplicable." One volunteer said that he couldn't pin down any significant changes, but concluded that the experience was interesting and fostered his belief in the idea that the individual is in touch with very little of reality. This man didn't have any interest in having the LSD experience again. He was satisfied that he had had it once.

The MAPS team identified three types of limited adverse reactions to the LSD experience. One participant said the experience itself was simply dreadful. He had apparently been given a double dose of LSD and felt terribly confused, very aggravated, and very miserable. He asked to have his wife by his side and to go home. Although he refused to talk about the specifics, he stated that lots of problems surfaced for him, noting that he had experienced psychological problems before he took the LSD. He didn't recall any life changes as a result of the experience, although he remarked that he was angry and fearful of having aftereffects. Nonetheless, he reported no flashbacks or persisting negative effects and concluded that he may not have been ready for the LSD. In the end he acknowledged that he may have learned something about himself.

In addition to the one overall negative LSD experience, two other types of adverse reactions presented themselves. First, a handful of respondents reported experiences that were generally positive but marked by significant negative aspects, ranging from experiencing physical pain to a temporary perceived loss of identity, to an inhospitable set and setting. In chapter 3 we also saw a number of such experiences described.

Some volunteers reported tremendous physical pain associated with the LSD experience. This included cramping and feelings of regression to the womb. Some experienced flulike symptoms, in which every bone in their bodies ached intensely. Another person reported that she lost her identity. (See chapter 6 for more such experiences.) She didn't have visions but she simply lost her sense of identity at the most intense part of the experience. Eventually, she had incredible visual experiences, which were quite thrilling and enabled her to perceive physical elements in a different way. She reported that she experienced the thin line between sanity and insanity. Nonetheless, it was one of the high points of her experiences and she loved it. The clergyman who became interested in consciousness studies was initially dissatisfied with the LSD experience. He complained the setting was nonconducive to spirituality and reported that, while under the influence of LSD, he experienced nothing more dramatic than nitrous-oxide-like laughter. In all five cases where negative elements were reported, they were resolved by the respondents who ultimately described their experiences as, on balance, positive.

The last type of adverse reaction involved negative long-term effects in the form of limited negative flashbacks. In twenty-six interviews where the interviewer attempted to specifically establish information about the nature and scope of flashbacks, the majority of respondents (nineteen out of twenty-six), did not report any. Two people reported negative flashbacks, four respondents reported flashbacks that they interpreted as beneficial, and one respondent described a neutral flashback. Of the two negative flashback reports, one came from a volunteer who may have been borderline schizophrenic and who had many symptoms before taking LSD. The other came from a respondent who had occasional flashbacks for perhaps six months. She reported looking at something that would appear to undulate—move about fancifully—and consequent feelings of losing control, which made her intellectually unhappy. However, she understood that these kinds of flashbacks could happen, and hers were not debilitating in any way.

At study's end the researchers concluded that within a nearly universally positive range, the nature, scope, and perception of the effect of the LSD experience on respondents' lives was relatively consistent.

While the goal of the original study was clearly not therapeutic, almost all respondents felt that the experience was a positive one. The team found minimal harm and perceived long-term benefits nearly forty years after individuals had participated in the LSD project.

The MAPS team drew several other conclusions of interest. First, they noted that Janiger modified the study conditions as he learned more about circumstances conducive to conducting his investigation. Rather than use a bench study where hypotheses were tested in rigid laboratory settings, Janiger chose to use a naturalistic method. This meant that the study design was qualitative, rather than quantitative, and evolving. The data on the artists is illustrative here. Once Janiger saw that artists could paint under LSD, he enhanced his procedures to make an art studio available for artists to demonstrate this capacity. Thus Janiger took information as it became available and used it to adapt his research model. This research approach fits into sociological notions of "the social construction of reality," in which knowledge about a social world is individually constructed and each individual's perception of experience is considered valid. When these perceptions are analyzed, the shared aspects of that knowledge form the basis for the researcher, in this case Janiger, to test emerging assertions within the current study context. To some degree, Janiger was a forerunner of the constructivist research approach.

Chapman and Alioto, two of the MAPS team members, point out a second noteworthy conclusion: The participants displayed remarkable intensity and emotional involvement in describing their experiences of forty years ago. While being interviewed by Chapman, the volunteers often were very cordial, relating colorful visions and insights they had from the most remote parts of their psyche. Their narratives were often very moving and vivid, as if the event happened just the other day. Alioto, who transcribed the participants' interview tapes, was also quite interested in how the passing of time and life's events had not dimmed the participants' memories of their LSD experiences. The respondents exhibited an emotional tone of excitement, wonder, intensity, and clarity. Their voices got louder as they remembered what they had seen, heard, or experienced. Many hadn't thought about the event for years and years, but they all asserted with passion and certainty that their memories were as sharp, clear, and vivid as if they had just had the LSD experience yesterday.

As Alioto points out, there was no social stigma, neither shame nor feelings of participating in something illegal, attached to the volunteers' LSD experiences. At the time of Janiger's study, LSD was seen as a medicine administered by a doctor. For many people the event was singular. They didn't have anyone in particular with whom they could discuss or compare it. Of course, this era of innocence didn't last. By the mid- and late 1960s, a good deal of now-discredited LSD research had found its way into the popular culture and was overpopularized. Mainstream society rejected LSD as inducing model psychoses or physiological damage.

In contrast, the MAPS team concluded that the moderate doses of LSD provided to volunteers in the context of Janiger's study caused little in the way of adverse reactions in the "normal" population. Even those volunteers who experienced initial adverse reactions ultimately went on to describe related benefits, such as changes in how they conducted their work, in their interpersonal relationships, or in their worldview. Based on the small sample of people interviewed, the team was not able to conclude if the experience was perceived as transformative, spiritual, or just deeply positive. They would have liked to know whether the LSD experience created any lasting behavioral changes, and if so, which and how.

The MAPS researchers concluded quite strongly that the evidence from their study "suggests that the FDA could feel comfortable about safety issues if it were to approve the administration of moderate doses of LSD to healthy human subjects by psychotherapeutically trained researchers working with the context of a scientifically meritorious research protocol." Moreover, they were convinced that the combination of Janiger's results and their findings constitute a clear call for further research into the beneficial effects of LSD. We end our chapter with their conclusion: "The preliminary findings [Janiger] made about the use of LSD in facilitating artistic creativity and about the nature of the LSD state as distinguished from its content provide a glimpse of fascinating research hypotheses that remain to be investigated with modern research tools and methodologies. This follow-up study confirms the lost opportunity suffered by science, medicine and religion when psychedelic research was shut down for essentially political, symbolic reasons. Research can be conducted safely, can generate important contributions to knowledge and can provide long-term benefits to a significant fraction of the subjects."

5

LSD, ART, AND THE CREATIVE PROCESS

FROM THE BEGINNING, many people suspected that LSD could heighten the creative capacity of the individual. Certainly, many participants in LSD studies report believing that their own creative abilities were enhanced. Moreover, some artists participating in Janiger's early study concluded that their LSD-inspired art had great aesthetic value—comparable to their other work. Controversy exists, however, as some artists and researchers have determined that LSD does not inevitably enhance creativity and can, in fact, impair the artists' technical execution and self-evaluation. Given such contradictory reports, further exploration into the relationship among LSD, art, and creativity could certainly prove rewarding.

But first, perhaps a few attempts to define difficult terms would be helpful. Of course, notions of *creativity* and *art* appropriately resist singular definitions, but for our purposes here, it may help to think of *creativity* as the capacity to create or produce, and *art* as one possible product of creativity. As many creations lack what most people would call creativity, we might add to our basic definition the qualities of imagination and originality, thus settling on a loose definition of creativity as the capacity to take existing materials and combine them in unusual ways to unique ends. The *creative process,* then, can be said to be the stages people go through as they engage in creative acts. Often the creative process is seen as a manifestation of some fundamental energy that is always accompanied by a sense of wonder, awe, amazement, the uncanny, the ineffable, the numinous. The Greeks characterized this process as a godlike source of artistic inspiration. From a psychoanalytical point of view, sexual energies are said to be sublimated to a creative drive.

Art is a still more controversial term. Early Greek critics defined art as the objective imitation of an external reality or truth; modern artists and critics tend to value art as the unique expression of subjective realities or truths. In any case, there does seem to be a distinction between the simply creative and the artistic. Janiger himself made a very real distinction between the two. To him, something that is artistic is inspirational. It has within it the potential for people to see and develop a variety of things that feed the individual's fantasies and whatever their definition of art is. In this sense, art is inciting while creativity—unique as a creative product may be—need not be, and artists are those creative people among us who dedicate their energies to reworking that which comes to them by inspiration, polishing and editing until it communicates to others.

The artist's most creative stance is to avoid becoming enmeshed in the conventional modes that delineate the world, and to keep a certain purity of perception—a kind of nonutilitarian reality common to children and adults with psychopathologies but uncommon in many of the rest of us, whose minds are fairly rigorously programmed to perceive an illusory world of unalterable reality. Historically, we can see that artists have often sought to change their mental states in order to facilitate and enhance their creative efforts. Clearly, these states can be called alterations of consciousness. These may occur spontaneously or can be brought about by manipulations of internal and/or external environments, and artists have commonly employed psychoactive substances such as alcohol, opium, hashish, nitrous oxide, or psychedelic drugs to achieve them. The use of these agents as facilitators could be seen as trivial or purely idiosyncratic if it were not for the extensive literature regarding their association with native and traditional folk art (see de

Rios 1974, 1977, 1981). Of course, in itself the use of these substances to alter perception is neither a sufficient nor necessary act to produce art. Their historical and widespread use by artists, however, suggests that the effects that are sought serve some function in the creative process, even if they don't necessarily manifest in an artistic product.

Research suggests that artists must pay a price for maintaining their creativity whether or not they employ psychoactive substances toward that end. Generally speaking, artists may not have the advantages of the "herd" and may live in a self-defined world. Creative individuals, according to psychologists, are most likely to be relative loners, have idiosyncratic ideas that they do not easily relinquish, and be strongly internally motivated and goal oriented. They may be unpredictable and prize new experiences. They may live uncomfortably close to the unconscious and to psychosis. Janiger considered artists as keepers of the Promethean flame, who risk the perilous journey to the heavens for the sake of bringing light to the rest of us that we may better see.

SCIENTIFIC STUDIES OF LSD AND CREATIVITY

Many scientists have investigated the effects of psychedelic substances on artistic creativity, and, as noted in earlier chapters, early research assumed that artists' behavior and work would result from an LSD-provoked "model psychosis." As early as 1955 a study of the effects of mescaline and LSD on four nationally-known visual artists revealed impairment of finger-tapping efficiency and muscular steadiness, but all were able to complete paintings. Pertinently, a panel of art critics judged the resulting paintings as having "greater aesthetic value" than the artists' usual work. They found that the lines were bolder and the use of color was more vivid (see Janiger and de Rios 1989).

Stanislav Grof, who began researching psychotherapeutic uses of LSD in 1960, recognized early on that the LSD experience caused colors to be typically perceived as very bright, penetrating, and explosive. He commented on the ornamentalization and geometrization of human faces, animals, and objects. Cohen, in his 1964 text *The Beyond Within,* described LSD's superlatives of intensity, luminescence, and saturation of color. Cohen also saw that under the LSD condition, people had the ability to exclude the clutter of random distractions and completely focus on the object before them. This is a total awareness—what has been called the "now moment." With LSD this timeless, selfless relationship with the object perceived—a relationship artists often experience, but which LSD intensifies—can be achieved by many. When this happens the object takes on a profound significance (as noted by many of Janiger's volunteer artists). As Cohen put it, "The separation between the one who sees and the seen vanishes."

Writing in 1966, Masters and Houston corroborated these early findings, arguing that some aspects of the psychedelic experience are important for artists because their awareness while under the influence of a psychedelic was profoundly different from their usual conscious waking states, dreams, or other familiar intoxication states. These writers found that the artists had greater accessibility to their unconscious; their ego boundaries were relaxed; their thought processes were fluent and flexible; their attention and concentration were intense or heightened; they had a high capacity for visual imagery and fantasy; they had an accelerated rate of thought; they had a seeming awareness of internal body processes and organs; they were aware of deep psychical and spiritual levels of the self; and they had the capacity for profound religious and mystical experiences. As creativity demands an openness to perceptions, LSD-like substances certainly seemed to be a fabulous tool for the creative process.

Yet as we have seen in earlier chapters, LSD affects each person differently, and psychologist Stanley Krippner, in his 1985 summary of nine major research projects on psychedelics and creative performance, makes it clear that there is no uniform psychedelic state. Silvano Arieti further argued in 1976 that while LSD enhances the primary creative processes, it impairs the secondary mechanisms needed to put the imagery to use. Krippner himself concluded that creativity is not automatically enhanced by psychedelics, and agreed with Arieti that technical execution often suffers. Furthermore, Krippner points out that the artist is not necessarily able to judge the value of the psychedelically inspired work while under the influence. It is clear that LSD can have a negative effect on motor performance and the concentration of naive subjects. Unlike Cohen, who described LSD's capacity to help artists exclude distractions and focus, some researchers have emphasized LSD's role as a means to decondition the individual, to throw open the gates that normally confine our perceptions to familiar territory. Such research—and some of the artists' comments below—suggest that LSD experiences may wildly enhance artists' creative potential without necessarily enhancing the mechanisms needed to harness that creativity toward artistic ends.

Yet it is also certainly true that LSD can have striking effects not only on artists' creativity but also on their work. In a study by Krippner of artists who were professionally committed to the creative life, he defined the term *psychedelic artist* as an artist whose work has been significantly influenced by the psychedelic experience and who acknowledged the impact of the experience on his work (see also Masters and Houston 1966). Interestingly, all of the artists who participated in Janiger's project said that LSD not only radically changed their style but also gave them new depths to understand the use of color, form, light, or the way these things are viewed in a frame of reference. Their art, they claimed, changed its essential character as a consequence of their experiences.

We don't really know how a person who uses LSD can combine his or her experience of sensory fields with emotion and memory to produce unusual imagery. Grof in his 1994 preface to *LSD Psychotherapy* wrote that LSD and other psychedelics function as "nonspecific catalysts and amplifiers of the psyche" that "do not have any specific pharmacological effects. They increase the energetic level in the psyche and the body which leads to manifestation of otherwise latent psychological processes." The "content and nature of LSD experiences are not artificial products of pharmacological interaction with the brain but authentic expressions of the psyche revealing its functioning on levels not ordinarily available for observation and study." The artist is the one who can transform these experiences into a creative work of art, music, or poetry.

JANIGER'S LSD ART PROJECT

The more than one hundred creative individuals—artists, writers, and musicians—who participated in a broader creativity study in which they took LSD invariably commented on the similarity of the LSD-induced state to what they felt might be an essential matrix from which the imaginative process derives. Almost all spoke of having gained a far greater insight into the nature of art and the aesthetic idea. Artistic productions—paintings, poems, sketches, and writings that stemmed from the experience—often show a radical departure from the artist's customary mode of expression. Paintings become more expansive and vibrant with an apparent disregard for likeness and conventional structural detail. The artists' general opinion was that their work became more expressionistic and demonstrated a vastly greater degree of freedom and originality.

The art project began serendipitously in 1954 when one of Janiger's early volunteers, a practicing professional artist, insisted on having some object to draw. His selection of a colorful deer kachina from Janiger's office shelf was a fortuitous choice. The doll had a symbolic resemblance to a human being. After his LSD experience the artist was very emphatic that it would be most revealing to allow other artists to go through this process of perceptual change. Janiger decided that a separate art project was worthy of exploration. This first artist was a teacher at a professional art institute and told many people about the project. Artists came in droves to ask Janiger if they could participate, but because Janiger did not want his research to be overwhelmed by an emphasis on art and creativity, he took pains to limit the number of volunteers in the substudy. By the close of the study, sixty practicing professional artists and forty writers and musicians had participated.

Janiger determined to include only trained artists. The artist had to be a professional, one who had been judged by peers, teachers, or others in the field. Some were artists who had made a reputation on their own by demonstrating proficiency and skills. Some were recommended by art schools. Janiger believed that LSD favored the prepared mind and believed that formal artists' training would best enable the group to benefit from the creative explosion during the LSD experience. Overall, reports show that these artists brought with them a natural sensitivity to beauty and order; a faculty of wonder; previous exposure to an environment that contained and encouraged creative work; formal organization of the creative impulse; training in mastering tools and craft; and the illumination or inspiration that in a flash composes the world into heightened and novel meaning.

The design of the study was simple and flexible. Janiger assumed at first that few artists would be able to paint under the effects of LSD. The artists were to be given a standard LSD dose and the expectation was that they would exhibit a significant lack of coordination. Janiger decided to use the same symbolically rich artifact, the deer kachina of the Pueblo Indians, that attracted the first artist. In a standard procedure, Janiger asked volunteers to paint or sketch the kachina doll at least once, about an hour after taking the LSD, in an art studio in Wilton Place. If he or she were willing, the artist was also encouraged to render the doll one hour before they ingested LSD, thus providing a map of the visual and perceptual directions that artists took in moving from one state of consciousness to another. In addition to these renderings, some artists drew self-portraits or attempted to capture their internal imagery while taking LSD.

For Janiger, mapping the volunteers' visual and perceptual changes was a most important way to look at LSD-inspired changes in perception and to understand the mechanism of creativity. Janiger hypothesized that by shifting perceptions the artists would shift their ability to extend their choices in how to render objects either in their environment or their inner images. Certainly, LSD facilitated a rush of new permutations, thoughts, and ideas, which served as a data bank of new information that the artist could draw upon. As the artists demonstrated, some people are gifted in organizing this flood of stimuli coming to conscious awareness at a fast pace and are able to hold on to the edge.

The artists concluded their participation in the study by responding to the same questionnaire sent to other volunteers thirty days after their LSD experience. Some of these responses are presented below.

Thirty-four years after the conclusion of his research, Janiger exhibited the art collection (and selected excerpts from the volunteers' narratives) in his home in Santa Monica, California, and received a fair amount of attention. While eight hundred invitations were sent out, some five thousand people responded.

Needless to say, a compelling question is whether the LSD-induced transformations in the volunteers' work represent enhancement or deterioration of the artistic product. We invite the reader's consideration, and offer fifteen samples of paintings and drawings from Janiger's substudy following page 118. In addition, appendix II presents poetry written at the end of the LSD experiences or a few days later. Naturally, researchers have drawn their own conclusions, as have the artists.

HERTEL'S ANALYSIS OF THE ARTWORK

During the seven years of the Janiger art experiment, 250 drawings and paintings were produced. These were examined in 1971 by Carl Hertel, then professor of art history at Pitzer College in Claremont, California, who undertook a stylistic assessment of the artwork. The following summary of his analysis is drawn from the catalog he wrote to accompany an exhibit of the work at the Lang Art Gallery at the Claremont colleges in 1971. There was an inherent difficulty in this kind of formal analysis because of the wide range of individual stylistic tendencies, in general, that characterize the work of contemporary Western artists. Hertel wrote that it would have been simpler to formally analyze the work of any tribal group that has definite traditional stylistic conventions than to analyze art produced under LSD.

The artists were a heterogeneous group whose stylistic tendencies included expressionistic, abstract-expressionistic, and nonobjective (expressing an ideal vision in the mind, separate from sensory perceptions). Nonetheless, Hertel found a striking homogeneity of stylistic effects in the works produced under the influence of LSD. Some of the artists were content with quick sketches of the kachina doll presented to them, while others were motivated to execute rather finished drawings and paintings. Hertel believed that it would have been a better design, not available to the study, to conduct longitudinal studies of individual artists before and after the experimental period, to evaluate the long-term effects of LSD on their work.

Hertel selected fifty-six items for detailed analysis, covering before and after samples of twenty artists in the deer kachina series. Another twenty-five items by eight artists were labeled series and represented free paintings and drawings done during the experimental period. They covered a wide variety of subject matter, including self-portraits, random drawings, and paintings. Of the eighty-one items, seventy-three were paintings done in various media and eight were drawings.

In analyzing the deer kachina series, Hertel established the following eight categories for classifying the works produced:

- The dominant style, if any, was identified to see whether the work was predominantly abstract, representational, or of another genre.
- Compositional characteristics were used to identify whether the composition was architectonic, a vignette, or of another style.
- Linear characteristics were examined to see whether the quality of line was nervous, angular, curvilinear, or of another form.
- Stroke characteristics were classified according to whether the predominant stroking was short and broad, broken, a flat field, or of another technique.
- Textural characteristics were examined to see whether the predominant textural quality was a heavy impasto (actual), illusionistic, or something else.
- Color characteristics were identified as noticeably local, arbitrary, brilliant, muted, or otherwise.
- Value characteristics were established to determine whether the use of lights and darks was strong in contrasts, close value, or another blend.
- Dimensional characteristics were also considered—whether the nature of the drawing and/or painting was suggestive of volume and mass, flat, two-dimensional, or otherwise.

Comparing the artists' work prior to and after ingesting LSD, Hertel found the most predominant changes were in the following categories: dominant style, color, line, and texture. When he focused on the representative changes in the dominant style category, he noted first that ten of the twenty artists were classifiable as predominantly representational in their customary approach to the subject matter. Their primary motive lay in representing the object as it presents itself to the eye. Of course, there was a great deal of individual variation within the representational approach.

Four of these ten artists changed their style under the influence of LSD to a noticeably expressionist one. Their primary interest lay in alterations of form, color, line, and medium. Within this group, the major tendency was to radically distort stroke and, therefore, medium and form. Image was retained in varying degrees. Three changed their style to a nonobjective one, replacing their focus on image with an interest in color and personal symbolism. One artist changed to a predominantly abstract style. The primary motive lay in the general reduction or simplification of forms and formal elements. In this case, the focus was shifted to a single part of the deer kachina. It might be noted that reduction is already a characteristic of the kachina style, but the reduction utilized by this artist and those in the following category exceeded what might be considered consistent with naturalistic representation.

Second, six of the artists were classifiable as normally predominantly abstract in the way they approached their subject matter. Under ordinary circumstances these artists made little or no attempt to provide pictorial representation. That is, their sensory experience was not perceivable by all observers. Of these six, three changed their style to a nonobjective one, two changed their style to being notably expressionist and engaged in radical distortions of composition and color, and one retained an essentially abstract style.

Third, two artists were classified as normally having distinctly expressionistic styles. In both cases, the predominant stylistic tendency was retained under the influence of LSD. However, changes in articulation of various formal elements, particularly line, were observed. (The work of the remaining two artists was stylistically ambiguous and therefore unclassifiable.)

As Hertel summarized, eight of the changes were to an essentially expressionistic style. Six were to a nonobjective one, which in many cases meant the expressionistic distortion of medium and color. He saw fourteen of the changes to a style in which the primary motive was an alteration of the representational image. Two of the changes were to a predominantly abstract style. Two other changes were ambiguous and unclassifiable. The changes followed a particular pattern: there was a movement toward alteration and fragmentation; there was an enlargement of the composition by means of focusing on parts rather than the whole; there was a movement with filling up the page; there was an intensification of color; there was a loosening up of the line to either a chiefly curvilinear (flowing) or sharply angular motive; and there was a general intensification of the textural properties of the medium used.

The results did not surprise Hertel. He suggested tentatively that although the work done under the influence of LSD was more interesting on a sensational level, it was not immediately clear that the individual artist—in the majority of cases—was able to produce aesthetically superior work during the period when the drug was operable. To be more specific, in a majority of cases a residual imprint of the artist's aesthetic preferences was retained. This was especially evident in choice of color and in technical facility. In those cases where technical proficiency appeared deficient in the pre-LSD state, a certain increase in the volunteer's ability to articulate or show confidence was seen due to the freedom apparently provided by the drug experience.

Hertel found a number of characteristics and commonly reported phenomena resulting from the LSD experience that had particular relevance to the question of creativity. In particular, there was greater freedom from prescribed mental sets and syntactical organization, and an unusual wealth of associations and images. Additionally, he found synesthesias, the sharpening of color perception, remarkable attention to detail, the accessibility of past impressions, memories, heightened emotional excitement, a sense of direct and intrinsic awareness, and the propensity for the environment to compose itself into perfect tableaux and harmonious compositions. The analysis also revealed perceptual changes in the artists that are indicative of those generally reported under the influence of psychedelics. The powerful global statements of the artists' work bears witness to these perceptual transformations. They can be examined at will (see insert following page 118) and serve as a prototype of the visual record of consciousness changes accompanying the creative process.

Hertel characterized the alterations in perception as follows:

1. Relative size, expansion. The artists' work tends to fill all available space and resists being contained within its borders, although the size of the image may vary.

2. Involution. Objects shrink down or fill less space. They become more compact or are imbedded in a matrix.

3. Alteration of figure/ground or shift to a circular viewpoint.

4. Alteration of boundaries. Figure and ground may be considered a continuum. The object tends to merge with the surroundings, with observer and observed not rigorously delineated, with less differential between the object and the subject.

5. Movement. The object or environment is in continuous movement with greater vibrancy and emotion.

6. Greater intensity of color and light.

7. Oversimplification. There is an elimination of detail and extraneous elements.

8. Objects may be depicted symbolically or as essences.

9. Objects are depicted as abstractions.

10. Fragmentation and disorganization.

11. Distortion.

Hertel himself did not pronounce a final judgement on whether the artwork he analyzed was enhanced or impaired by LSD. The artists themselves, however, had no reluctance to speak their minds.

THE ARTISTS SPEAK OUT

Contrary to Janiger's initial expectation, most artists do find it possible to exercise some technical proficiency, with varying degrees of success, under the influence of LSD. To Janiger's surprise, he also found that artists gradually became more adept working under the influence of LSD. They somehow found a way to draw inspiration from the LSD state for the creation of art and were increasingly able to control the physical expression of their subjective vision. The artists who were most able to represent their subjective LSD experiences in their art were those who had most developed their technical abilities so that they had the rigor to bring back to consensual reality their artistic vision. One artist stated that this experience was "more creative than a dream, more original than that of a madman's vision."

Nevertheless, as Hertel and others have noted, the psychedelically inspired artistic products are not, ipso facto, superior to those performed in ordinary states of consciousness. On the other hand, these artistic productions are not, ipso facto, inferior either. The artists' narratives and follow-up questionnaires reveal that the works are often judged by the artists to be more interesting or even aesthetically superior to their usual mode of expression. In many cases, the artists felt that the LSD experience produced some desirable lasting change in their understanding of their work, which continued to influence the form and direction of their artistic development. Some noted that a so-called confessional or disorganized phase followed, which may represent a creative crisis in which artists struggle to maintain their traditional approach until they reach another level of integration and expression.

These metamorphoses all contributed to the artists' convictions that they were able to create new meanings in an emergent world. Overall, the artists reported that in their LSD experiences they had gained the ability to generate original insights, fresh perspectives, and novel, creative form.

From the artists' follow-up questionnaires Janiger excerpted a group of narrative accounts of the experience that were displayed in the 1985 art exhibit. In this section some of the artists' diverse experiences are presented. Many of their statements are paraphrased by the author when not presented in direct quotes.

D.V.

I have learned for myself that art is more nearly allied to man's pre-human state and that science is the most human of man's activities, not art. I have less tolerance for what I might call the pseudo-human and pre-human in our midst. I am more than ever convinced that man must use his reason to be human. There was nothing in the LSD experience to change my atheist viewpoint except to reinforce my belief that revelation is a psychological phenomenon.

S.R.

I went immediately to work upon arriving at the studio. The color I used became alive on the brush. All self-consciousness, value and judgment disappeared. Paint became like shining liquid metal and ink like expanding jewels. I was capable of attention only in the area of my brush and it seemed impossi-

ble to attend to the composing of an area larger than two or three square inches. The excitement of the materials and the surfaces became overwhelming. After working for a certain amount of time, I became more conscious of space and area and application of paint became like great explosions, strokes always radiating from a center, then trailing or swirling off to radiate from another. The brushes seemed too small, and I moved to a three-inch house brush. Before long I was dipping into the paint cans with my hands and pouring colored inks from the bottles. Color and form vibrated and moved with the music being played and waves of joy and excitement flooded through me. The universe manifested itself in the spreading of ink on soft paper and color fusing became like the exploding gasses on the surface of the sun.

Sheet after sheet of paper was used, chip, matte, and illustration boards —anything I could get my hands on. Subject matter began to enter the work, but changed with the new suggestion of each new stroke. The themes of sunflower, flying horse, playful dragons and exploding flowers dominated in the avalanche of suggestion.

Q.R.

This artist was very curious and enthusiastic to experience something new. He was sure there would be no danger involved and no lasting after effects. He saw some of the pictures of the kachina doll leaning against the walls, done by other artists, and the perceptual distortions began. He set up the easel and placed the now-famous kachina doll at eye level, to paint an impression of the artifact. He had already ingested the appropriate LSD dosage for his weight. Here is what he wrote during the experience:

I am involved with space, volume, tension factors—the usual concerns that one has when creating a picture, using negative space to relate with the object. I call the sketch finished and sit down on the couch to wait—I feel full headed, vaguely dizzy but not unpleasantly so. My face feels thicker, as if I am becoming aware of the outer extremity of myself. I look in the mirror—my face looks translucent, nothing dramatic. I close my eyes to guess the time lapse of three minutes. I check my watch, one minute gone. I think I'll paint the doll now. My pen seems to rush ahead of my thoughts, the reverse of usual sensations. At 2:00 P.M., two hours after LSD ingestion, I *sketch another doll. No distortion of image. I only am interested in doing a quick sketch. My hand bearing down on this paper with this pen seems unconnected to me, or the paper, lovely sensation, eyes feel washed. I'm smiling. No image shifting, distortion, just marvelous clarity. Color is clean, clear, eyes so cleaned. Objects startlingly there. I see space. It shimmers like heat waves, as exciting to see as objects, all separate, all belonging. I belong.*

I feel fatuous, like a bodiless grin, smiling a ribbon of pleasure around all I see, around everythingness. At 2:28 P.M., I feel so happy, listening to a classical music piece which doesn't demand my attention as usual. . . . Lots of undulation—I sketch the doll again. Why doesn't it change? Only two-dimensional changes. Pictures undulate, walls undulate. 3D objects when I look directly are immobile. At 3:40 P.M., the Kachina doll still appears the same. I throw up in the toilet. There is the smell of vomit all around.

He became fascinated with negative spaces, which seemed to have an entity as exciting as objects, akin to the concern with them in painting but inexpressibly more acute.

These negative spaces became objects, dark spaces between objects became objects of great mystery. Purple and deep red that no pigment could achieve in tonal depth or intensity. Juxtaposition of red and green seemed to have a more heightened intensity of hue, and for me, were more subject to animistic perception. The surface on which black and white pictures were painted undulated as well as the images upon them. They didn't shift. This set me to wondering if the heightened senses of smell, color, form and sound isn't so entirely staggering to our usual habit of perceiving that we lose control of the faculty to relate, there being too much going on all at one time.

When he looked at the black-and-white pictures there were not as many other factors involving the sight sensorium. Consequently, he found less breakdown of the faculty to relate objects and negative shapes. He became interested in hallucinating and optical illusion. If hallucinating is determined by seeing new objects, which are not there at all, he reports that he didn't hallucinate in that sense. However, if hallucination means to see actual objects seemingly performing in a manner one knows is imagined or impossible, such as a rearrangement, undulation or intensified color perception, that is another matter. He asked: "How different is this from optical illusion?"

In some ways this encounter disappointed the artist, who found himself torn between an eagerness to experience fully and the desire to remain detached enough to retain a reasoning consciousness that could record accurately what he experienced. While he did not hope to prove any preconceived ideas, he wrote that he must have had a subconscious need to retain his most conscious self-concept—a need he ultimately found self-defeating in light of his simultaneous, staggering determination to see himself performing his task (painting the kachina doll) during LSD. It was a large, imposing, exciting, fascinating, enjoyable, and humbling experience, so much so that his determination to impose his rational thinking processes upon it loom suggestively in his mind as superegocentric and overly motivated.

The artist wrote that he should like to take LSD again in a quiet room, white and plain, to see if he would discover some psychological insights that largely escaped him the first time, once removed from the stimulus of color and an art experiment. He wrote that he was too strongly motivated toward a specific task and was not able to focus on his own psychological issues. His usual feeling of kinship with people and things, subjects and objects, seemed to be unaltered, only intensified and confirmed. This first experience was beyond personal emotional or intellectual concepts, yet still a part of it. He wanted to lovingly embrace the universe as it correspondingly embraced him. This was the essence of the unself-consciousness of his experience.

This sense of harmony with and belonging to remained with the artist to the end.

When we got home, the living room seemed much larger, the chairs stood out as if suspended in some eternal isness. The sense of empty space was different. Space was an entity in itself and personal as much in my awareness of objects. When I got into bed, I was aware of feeling different than usual. Ordinarily I have a tingly delicious feeling of a total body related to everythingness. This evening after LSD I felt myself as a shape resembling a four pointed starfish. I fell asleep smiling and awoke at 1:00 A.M. to notice the louvered windows were still moving.

Despite the artist's belief that his experience failed to produce psychological insights, his report is unusually eloquent in describing LSD's capacity to interact with and unlock the psyche.

I imagine that a person coming to the experience with built-in hostility toward his environment and including interpersonal relationships cannot but view with alarm the animistic quality of the experience. Seeing an increased threat when usually perceived objects seem to take on the capacity of moving about? If a man or woman who was overly attached to their own beauty were to view their face, as I saw mine, aging and deeply lined, might not this impose a sense of horror? LSD offers a key to just these insights into the personality, which might otherwise be locked in a subtle self-hiding process and the degree of intensity of their reactions as evoked under LSD would serve as a key or clue. LSD certainly imposes a demand on one's attention independent of their ability to process, evaluate or relate back to the structured self. A short cut. As to whether LSD is a key to the origins of the creative impulse, I am clouded over that. Freud's concept indicates that the artist uses his media to express fantasy in a manner which takes a new form of reality an image of reality and as a result he is able to enjoy the catharsis of escaping the censorship of first cause.

Until such day as we come to know what is implied in the term Human Being, all the arts will continue to be our substitute body, the imagery of reality instead of the tools by which we may locate, instruct and confirm our humanity, the tools we could employ as recorders of our growth toward that illusive perfection of perception, directly and not in the manner of abstracting the essence of our most inner truth.

O.A.

This artist rendered the kachina doll before LSD took full effect.

I am again struck by a certain restraint and rigidity in my drawing. Will the LSD liberate my hand so that I may achieve a kind of free and easy expression as opposed to what may be called rather "stiff?"

[At 10:40 a.m.:] I'm now very high. I'll try another sketch now. The colors seem to have taken on an iridescence—except that the feeling is that of evanescent iridescence. [At 10:55 a.m.:] I was going to make a sketch before but never got around to it. Will do so now. I almost got to do the drawing, but it was a little difficult and I felt there were other sensations to report. One is that I seem to be very amused by what's happening. I know my senses are being distorted but there is still this underlying core of reasonableness, almost standing aside and observing all of this. With respect to the drawing and the Kachina doll, although I am conscious of these distortions of vision, I do not see any basic change in the doll. If I am unable to draw it, it is not because I can't see it accurately enough through all this fluidity—it is because physically I almost feel incapable of holding on to the pen and making it do what I want it to. Now I'm going to try again, that is, to draw. Kind of amazing. I can't seem to hold on to any thought or concept for any appreciable length of time. It's almost as if I lose the sentence in mid-stream. At times, there seems to be a wedding of the senses. I can't tell whether I'm seeing something or tasting something. [At 11:15 A.M.:] It looks like I'll never get to that drawing. Keep on feeling it is necessary to report my sensations. I would say that the distortions are becoming so strong that they are indeed hallucinatory—to say the least.

In terms of the drug as it affects one's creativity, I would say that it doesn't make me any more or less creative than I already am. It doesn't liberate thoughts that were supposedly deep down inside just bursting to come forth. However, it seems to me that even if I am coherent long enough that whatever comes out will probably be distorted. I am conscious of that basic core of reason and the "critical observer" beneath the flux.

I thought that in my drawing, there would be some strange new force guiding my hand but such isn't the case. My intellectual resources stay the same but because of the LSD they will undergo some distortion. I don't feel any more creative than normal. If there seems to be a change in my drawing, it's not intentionally—or because of a basic change of perception. I can still perceive what is correct or should be correct, but I can't stay coherent long enough to put it down that way. So in the case of the drawing, the apparent freedom isn't really that at all. It's just an inability to put it down correctly. I can't even seem to hold onto the pen long enough.

Just this constant state of flux in all of the senses. The culling of hidden creative resources, this the LSD doesn't do for me. There is no great creative insight. Just distortions. I don't feel any more creative. With LSD the reality is always there but going through a constant changing flux.

Q.B.

This volunteer was curious to experience a new emotional and visual sensitivity and gives a rare, sustained portrait of the degree to which LSD can both concentrate an artist's awareness and make concentration on a task impossible. He brought a large selection of pastels with which to draw the kachina that had been placed on the table in front of him. After five minutes he became less interested. He did not want to do a picture of the kachina doll, or anything else, for that matter. He felt a fluttering sensation inside his body, like a heart flutter. He was drawing the picture badly, due to a lack of interest. Textures and colors throughout the LSD experience were of dominant interest to him. He started a second drawing of the kachina doll at someone's urging. His attention was arrested—which plagued him for the rest of the experience. The box of pastels became a thing of such monumental beauty, a container of the most fantastically glowing colors. For him, the selection of one color became almost impossible. However, once he did make the selection, the putting down of a line on the rough drawing paper became so utterly pleasurable and an experience of such intense beauty that to follow with another line was almost a negation of the first. The instant that it took him to form a line became prolonged. It was possible for him to see the line form, to watch the pastel form on the paper, to see it leave the stick and become the line.

It was like being a first hand witness of creation. No artist would be able to create if he saw his medium form itself into the art which he was working.

Even his hands became things of interest. They had become literally smeared with pastel. The colors overlapped, not mixing as we usually see them. When a red overlapped yellow, instead of seeing an orange color of some sort, it was perfectly possible to see the yellow underlying the red. The colors had transparency and depth. He felt that he could have measured the depth of them on his hands had he so desired.

He went out for a walk on the street. On crossing Wilton Place, the textures of the street and sidewalks came into an entirely new sharp focus. Ordinary cracks appeared to be canyons. The surface of the walks was pitted and pocked. The concrete reflected colors from all surrounding areas, such as buildings, automobiles, lawns, and so forth. Just walking on these surfaces became a magnificent experience for him.

On the walk he became very much aware of the fact of his sex, that he was a man and therefore he was different from perhaps half the people on the street. It was an awareness and consciousness that stuck with him pretty much for the duration of the day. He was conscious of the breadth of his shoulders, of the depth of his chest. He could feel the muscles of his arms and legs working as he walked. He became and remained noticeably sex-conscious, not in an erotic way but merely aware of his own sex and sexual areas.

Colors were no longer merely exterior reflections of light. They were a part of him—or he was a part of them. When he studied a color, warm as well as cool by this time, he felt he was seeing a new depth of color. He became the color. He identified himself with the color; it became an absolutely personal thing. He experienced the LSD as waves of sensation, which became less and less intense as time wore on.

The LSD helped tremendously to relieve inhibitions I had had in my art work. It taught me the value of the impressionistic approach to my art. This impressionistic area of thinking now enters into my work whether it is realistic or abstract. I feel I can sit down now, relax, and evaluate the true nature of the problem to be solved. I can put down a precise aesthetic answer to the problem, which rarely is accepted by my profession. So many rigid rules are taught in schools. So many taboos are self-imposed by the artist himself because of prejudices and jealousy. This LSD helps release the artist from these bonds. I had previously been of the formal school of realism. I have now learned to express myself symbolically.

D.I.

It was when I began the third drawing that energy suddenly poured through me in a joy so overpowering that I cried and these emotions continued to surge through me for the rest of the afternoon. At what I think was the peak of the reaction of the LSD, I knew with certainty that the previous drawings were immature and bad art, that the one I was working on was very good, and that the next ones would be equally as good.

I can't emphasize strongly enough how conscious I was of the joy in drawing at this time. My whole being enjoyed the sensual experience of applying chalk, of enjoying the resultant beauty of the markings on the paper, of slowly and lovingly retracing the strokes and then of being caught up in the desperate longing to be able to continue remembering in my future activities that the truth of creative expression is being able to get out of my own critical way, with full awareness that I could allow my creative side full rein.

C.L.

I feel artists should have this LSD experience to free preconceived ideas of art and facilitate their ability to express themselves. It gives greater understanding and feeling of the creative experience. My creative process was intensified by LSD.

L.Y.

I perceived all visual detail more precisely. I saw a fuller range of color than I customarily do, I noticed things which have been familiar for years but which were unperceived. The two paintings done under the LSD are painting of my emotions. The one in which the horns remain is not unlike the beginnings of paintings I have done in the past, but the abstraction embodies a wild flight of emotion unlike anything I have ever done as a painter. I recall scribbling it compulsively and it contains a high level of emotion. This is the only measure I can suggest, but I do feel that the whole LSD episode was dominated by an access to emotion greater than I normally have.

C.K.

What I saw can't be explained in words. It is as simple as that. I only hope that my paintings will show a little of this vision. And if just a little comes through the surface, I will be quite satisfied.

In a sense, this story is not complete. The hero should have returned to his studio to paint the greatest masterpiece of the century. But this did not happen. That night, after returning to my studio, I finished the pastel I began that afternoon and did two more, working into the early hours of the next morning. The next day I finished a painting I had been working on for a week, unifying it in a matter of two hours. What had happened? The answer lies in the area of experience. I had witnessed the unity of the Universe and could now paint with this knowledge. This knowledge might prompt the subtlest change in line or color or attitude on my part, but it is just this kind of fine adjustment that can make a painting "work" in terms of color or movement or meaning. It means that I have adopted a new, higher criteria. It doesn't mean that magic will gush from my brush, but rather that I will paint and paint some more until the painting arrives at what I want it to be.

L.C.

I believe that artists should have this experience to break through the barrier of adjusted feelings, to fling open visual, tactile and emotional doors that get standardized, to set up standards of visual experiences of such intensity as to force the habit of creative and bold search. LSD speeds up change so that it can be observed. It intensifies and magnifies to show sources. It eliminates the conceptual that is not incorporated into the emotional. It eliminates competitiveness and the search is lyrically that of an emotional language. LSD verified for me the essence of art as endless change. Also, that you never lose anything in a painting, only change and purify it.

R.K.

Most artists work in terms of systems or periods or perspectives. LSD helps clarify the current approach. LSD helps pose new "what if" problems artists are always asking. LSD beautifully helps show relationship between two dissimilar objects. LSD helps synthesize. An artist compresses reality. LSD helps see the phrase or picture in its most complex and succinct form. LSD helps act as a standard to the artist to see if he's committed enough of himself to the work at hand.

LSD helps the artist to know himself, which is the main thing. It helps us experience more of the work we see or hear, so with LSD we might get closer to the actual chaos the artist is trying to fix when he creates. Also, a trained disciplined artist can not distort or break rules, which is one of the essences. LSD helps you extend. No, you don't forget rules or form, but you extend beyond the limit they have on you.

It made me realize I wanted to explore the limits of form. It gave me confidence to extend and push beyond safe water, knowing if I got in over my head, intuition could help. I believe now that intuition is a valuable tool of the craft. I am not afraid to use it. I believe how that it will help. It sees more than

I, remembers more. It is usually right. With form and discipline, you can copy. That's easy. But add intuitive feelings and you create.

L.R.

Each one of us is born into a community whose habits, customs, etc. become ours. These legacies of society can become a real burden or hindrance to a creative attitude. It seems that our social behavior is governed by what is wrong or right. We judge everyone and everything with an end aim of perfecting our deductions by what is called having sound judgment. In art, these ideas are reflected in our thinking, by passing judgment. This means in our approach to art, we have preconceived ideas about what the end product should be. Words seem to build a wall between us, and our resources. The emphasis seems to be on the results of the past, instead of discovery. We work backwards when in truth, original experience exists for us every moment. Suspending one's judgment is not a widespread habit in this country. The scientific attitude lies in this difference and not what is so called good or bad. They are invested in the behavior of factors, which can be predicted by various means and devices. Until the scientist abandoned the idea of purpose, they couldn't develop sufficient causes in the procedure of their action to develop anything at all. Therefore, things get their character from the relationship in which they perform. As far as our perception of time, and mass and distance, they tell us nothing about the true nature of things.

This artist believed that we have to unlearn some things we believe to be self-evident truth, a form of deconditioning.

Our destiny is unknown; security prevents experimentation; the old way feels right. Failure is not due to lack of effort, but is due to making the wrong move. We cannot experience the same thing.

L.B.

There was love in everything. The brushes, the paper, the paints, they were all alive with good, happy vibrations. . . . There was a tremendous feeling of joy and love surrounding me. As I painted, I felt a closeness to my materials that I had never experienced before, as if they were joined, every color vibrated. All were intensified. It didn't seem to matter what color I used, or where my brush stroke traveled. As soon as the color reached the paper, or the stroke was completed, it became right, harmonious and meaningful, part of the plan. There was such pleasure and joy in every stroke. The thought became the action in a conscious fluid stroke. When I cried, the tears flowed through the brush onto the face of the girl I painted. My tears were her tears.

C.A.

I came into a room here with a mountain of complexities and in a short hour, I was reduced down to the essence and essentials of painting for me. COLOR. Right there. No doubt about it. Just color. No form, no line. Space was not important, ideas could go to hell! All that began to exist was color, pure and brilliant. It was like walking into a room with a cobweb full of ideas, doubts, thoughts about painting, and then just leaving them all way behind you and being reduced down to the essence of it all. The "why" of painting. And, this was plenty in itself. In fact, it became everything.

It was a complete education in itself. I think I found out what color was to me. Or what I was to color. I felt fresh, pure and whole. In that I felt as a child. Perhaps I saw as a child might see color. I do know that I saw color like I had never seen it before. It was like seeing should be. All my so-called adult learned things just left. In seeing color in its own being, on its own terms, I think I found some of myself. The LSD has changed my seeing. Probably my person too.

I have seen with new eyes of what canvas looks and feels like, and is. What brushes do, and how paint can deliciously swim and flow onto a canvas. In LSD, the learned part of you just leaves and you are left with just yourself. Then you just do what you have to do. There is no conscious awareness about your composition or what you are saying of anything except what you have to do. You just do it and it seems right.

Reflecting on his experience further, he wrote the following:

I was a participant in a creative research project of LSD. I am a painter and I had planned to paint under the influence of LSD. I had no idea if I would paint or if I would want to. But I did feel a responsibility to do so, since this was the reason I was given LSD. Before taking it, I did a reasonable self-portrait of myself in pencil for the purpose of seeing a "before" and "after" result. I started to feel the effects about an hour after I was given LSD. The first thing I noticed was the intensity of color. Color hues became very brilliant. It was like seeing color for the first time. The intensity of the color became so intense that it flickered. I began to see the room as patches of brilliant color. Outside there was no negative space, in pictorial terms, as everything was positive. The space between things was as positive and as real as things or objects. Some objects like my hands flowed with a slight blue-purple fringe around them. Movement, like when one moves one hand in front of your face became more than just a blur. Because I could see more than a blur. It was like seeing a photograph of movement, being able to see the hand in two different places at once. Space was different, but I can't explain how. I wondered how it was possible to draw. Why draw, in fact. I had no motivation to draw or paint, all I wanted to do was to just to sit and to look. Just be. My whole body felt good. Every time I concentrated on something, color would dominate me, and I would just look at color. I begin to see that I was bathing in a world of color that I have never seen before. It was not the color of the object but just the color itself. That was enough. I wished I could have seen no objects, no anything except color. Sometimes I did. I could see how one could be thrown into a complete abstract world of fantastic color, void of object, associations, void of everything except color. There was a certain amount of special distortion. For the first time, I think I understood color. Understood it for itself. Since I came here to paint, I thought about it, but it seemed such an inadequate, hopeless and meaningless thing to do at this time. Besides I had no desire to do anything except look. I tried to draw, but a pencil or a line wasn't enough because there was too much color. I did draw a few lines and began to appreciate just the line for itself. I didn't want the line to represent anything because it alone was fascinating. I was afraid the paint I brought along would not be brilliant enough to satisfy me. I felt there were two colors now: 1) the color I saw on objects and 2) the color that was in my tubes and the color of my mind, which I was seeing for the first time. All of a sudden I understood Indian color, Mexican color, color of primitive cultures, the color of South America.

I attempted another self-portrait (no 2), because the other self-portrait I did, prior to the taking of LSD, frankly looked ridiculous. It was not me. I didn't look like that, nor feel like that. I looked absurd and a fake. That portrait looked false to me. No 2 which is the second self-portrait, felt better, because it felt like everything around me was just intense color and I was almost blinded by it. I attempted another self-portrait. I tried to be somewhat realistic. I even looked in the mirror, but my nose became orange, and an ocean of blue began swimming into my check. Line and pencil just didn't satisfy me, because color was so prominent. I guess I knew by this time that any kind of representation was impossible at this point.

At this point, I started on one of my canvases. I don't know what time it was, as I didn't care. It was not important. I had some difficulty in motivating myself to action of any sort. I reworked the first self-portrait I did before I took LSD. It needed colors and it got them. At this time, around 3:00 P.M., I was really getting into the swing of painting. When I looked at my brushes, the tips of them glowed with the various pigments that they had been dipped in. Complementary color really jumped. It breathed. All color was more intense. Analogous color also jumped and became alive. It flickered too. The yellow glowed the most, so I selected that. Others were single blocks of color. It had to be by itself, pure, and in no shape. At this point, I ran out of paper (after doing nine paintings and in canvas). I painted on my paint box. I painted on the back of my data sheet. I painted part of the wall yellow.

My painting went from complex to simple. Painting simply reduced itself down to its essence. For me, on that day, it was color. On another day, it might be line or shape or space. It was a complete education in itself. I think I found out what color was to me. I felt fresh, pure and whole. I do know that I saw color like I had never seen it before. It was like seeing should be. In seeing color in its own being on its terms, I think I found some of myself. Three of the pictures I did are the most honest statement I have ever made. The LSD has changed my seeing. Probably my person, too. I have seen with new eyes of what canvas looks and feels like and is. What brushes do, and how paint can deliciously swim and flow into a canvas. I recognized under LSD that a painter has two forces that are in constant play in the process of painting or drawing. One is the learned. Your trained hand, how your hand can move and make forms because it knows how to make those forms. It is just trained. The other force is what is not learned. Perhaps it is you or your emotion. In LSD, the learned part of you just leaves and you are left with just yourself. Then you just do what you have to do. There is no conscious awareness about your composition of what you are saying, of anything except what you have to do. You just do it and it seems right. Perhaps when we normally paint, without LSD, the conscious and unconscious are in constant play or *the intellect and the emotional are in play. In LSD there is no play. You just paint. There is no struggle, worry, because it just flows out. And it seems right and valid. Today it still looks valid because I know did it honestly yesterday. The fact that I did it is enough of a validity. When I painted under LSD, color became the most important thing. It was reduced to its essence, itself. There was no compromise, no reference. The color alone was enough. Almost too much.*

The LSD was a most rewarding and revealing experience. Today I see things differently than I did yesterday. It in some ways could be termed a mystical or religious experience. I feel in accord now, more than ever, with the world I live in. My vision is sharper. It has changed me. I appreciate now the worlds of other painters more because before I had naturally liked painters who I felt were close to my world. LSD opened up other painters, e.g., Matta, Parker, Gorky, Rothko, etc.

V.L.

At 10:00 A.M. the volunteer, an artist and physician, took five LSD pills. He experienced a moderate subjective vertigo. Progressively he became less coordinated, had a shortened attention span, and he became more acute in his visual and auditory perceptions. By noon he gave up trying to paint. He was a Sunday painter, and mixing pigments was too much for him to concentrate on. He started to write. At 4:00 P.M. he started a drawing. He shut his eyes and was overwhelmed with a beautiful unfolding colored vision, which started as an afterimage of what he had been looking at. The lovely colors, which flowed in all directions, were mostly formless. He found himself very concerned with his bodily perceptions. He flexed and extended his arms, hands, feet, legs, and so on. He stared at his body and the room, and he seemed to use his body. The room itself was a reference point, a link to reality. He tried to paint again. That was no good. He tried clay, but it was too much effort. He started to draw. Then he put away his paints and packed up. When he was painting, he reported that he was too physically weary to hang on to the paintbrush. He was very nearly unable to control the pen. Fear struck him that he would forget this experience. He was too shaky and tremulous to tear the paper. He felt that if he put down the pen he would not be able to pick it up again.

F.L.

LSD is a great aid in finding one's own nature. To understand the meaning of the symbols they use, by studying their work not painted under LSD as well as painting done under LSD. To enrich them and their views, to paint with respon- sibility to themselves and the viewers. LSD can show the ordinary person a greater view of things, which may make them more appreciative of art forms and manners previously passed over without consideration. It gave more pur- pose to my role as an artist. It concentrated my ability to sum up the essence of a subject.

L.G.

For me, LSD opened up a whole new world of creative possibilities both in art and in my life. I became more daring and more willing to venture into the unknown, into the mysterious. It helped free me from the pressures of false reality, which imprisoned a heightened sense of imagination. Again, I would say it stimulated my imaginative reaction to life. I began to create a mytho- logical world of my own out of shapeless materials. Under LSD, I focused for a while on the Kachina doll, but then I became the child with the terrifying bur- den of the fear of isolation—a painfully separate person with nothing to lean on. That was the beginning of faith for me. For in faith, I was no longer alone.

A.R.

After I was on, the Kachina doll itself was like a dead wooden thing, a bent hol- low dead figure with decorations and no meaning. Like nothing. I sort of painted a creature that was perhaps this doll's God. Alive, fiery, pagan, evil, and very dumb. Anyhow, to hold a brush while on LSD was something else— like it was a magic wand and I could create any kind of image I wanted. Each stroke was an experience which added up to the total painting, but to me it was not the finished painting that was important but much more important was the joy in painting itself.

A.V.

I started to paint with red paint and for a while I did not consider time as existing. I also had no idea of myself as existing. I reacted to an object when I came in contact with it. There was no separation between an object and myself. I was everything around me, and when I moved, my surroundings moved to fit me.

O.Y.

I had the feeling of being very suggestible and everything seemed of equal importance and validity. I felt no desire to follow a single theme or idea or even concern myself with concepts or styles of drawing. Therefore, the drawing became an organic entity recording the thoughts and influences existent at the time of the drawing. I experienced a sensation of the nearness of the now-now.

Q.L.

LSD has opened my willingness to let imagination play a greater role. It has led me to take a stronger position vis-a-vis the world of philosophic attitudes, thus revealing greater commitment to my work. Aside from the revelation of beauty that is involved, the deeper value of LSD is the re-evaluation of life that takes place and a relocation of one's role in society.

H.L.

I began the process of picking up the brush, and as my hand moved in the direction of where the brush was lying, I watched it, and it was a real hand thing, and it reached the brush and the hand became the brush, the brush became the hand. I put my fingers inside the handle and the old ink and hairs, feeling and feeling as the brush felt back at me. It was wet with ink-wash. As it touched the paper, more beautiful shapes and Things happened, just happened. I saw the grain of the paper, into it, around it, and it was touched by me as well as my touching it. I have used line in drawing for years. With LSD the line became a thing in itself as I made it. I would look at a thing or object like the doll and see many things too quickly. I mean too quickly to catch them, but not too quickly to see them. Then I would attempt to draw, to try to express what I saw in the object and all my involvement wound up on the paper and the brush and the ink, etc. So I tried not looking at the paper or the brush but at the object. Then I was involved with how the brush felt in my hand and how my hand felt ad infinitum.

Q.M.

I feel that artists should have this experience. It will give them greater aware-
ness of themselves and to life. An artist must travel through all the doors of
this earth and LSD is one of the greatest doors to perception I have witnessed.
Regarding if LSD can be used as an approach to understanding or enhance-
ment of creativity, if one's mind is capable of leaving its own shell he may trans-
pose himself into that of the artist's work he is seeing or listening to—if he is
moved by the experience, then he will understand the content of the work and
probably touch upon the artist's identity as well. LSD did not make me more
creative—however it did open up new avenues for me to do further research
in color as well as black and white. I have always believed that a truly creative
being is always high—childlike and yet philosophical. With my first introduc-
tion to LSD, I found my already hypersensitive being become kinetically more
so. A new dimension opened itself before me.

Visual artists were not the only creative people affected by LSD.
Musicians and writers, too, had very powerful experiences.

R.O., a psychologist and writer

Having always had difficulty with myopia as well as limited color vision, I now
found myself describing color and form in a most unusual detail. I was able to
look into the heart of a blossom and see the most minute changes and alter-
ations in structure and movement. It was simply a feast of the senses and as I
turned to observe people and broader aspects of the scene I was enraptured
by a series of tableaux which were similar to paintings. I observed . . . a
Breughel painting in which the colors and shapes astounded me by their clar-
ity. I felt a great surge of perceptual power.

Q.S., a musician

An accomplished composer and musician, he commented on how he
experienced music under the LSD experience.

There were a lot of subjective reactions that I had that I don't feel I could . . .
explain which have to do with the significance of the music. I brought along,
at the invitation of Dr. Janiger, certain compositions, which I thought would

yield up various kinds of reactions. I brought a Schoenberg record, a piece which had disturbed me by my total lack of comprehension of it. I brought along a late Beethoven quartet, the holy song of thanksgiving of the convalescent to the deity. I brought along a Bach chorale prelude to see what would happen to the perception of the polyphonic texture of various melodies going at the same time in pure harmonic framework. I brought along a work by a master composer of the twentieth century, whose work had meant a great deal to me—Bartok—his last string quartet.

And, I brought along a Dylan Thomas record to see what would happen to my perception for a conceptual kind of art, since music deals in a kind of super-conceptual framework which can't be diluted easily into words. I thought that the problems and the results that I would get from listening to that music would be quite different than what would happen if I listened to a poem, which dealt with concepts and verbal things.

The experience lasted almost fourteen hours. In the twilight of the experience, in the late evening when I was listening to some things, one—the Bartok quartet which instead of being divided into movements, occupied one whole side of an LP with no bands in-between. With this and the Dylan Thomas poem, read by myself, called a "Winters Tale"—both of them had presented problems to me in the previous workaday reality of grasping their meaning. And I was most struck [by] . . . my span of attention, which is something that interests me both as a performer and a music lover, which is something I am despite the fact that I'm professionally involved in it. I was most struck with the fact that this Bartok quartet which has a span of some twenty five minutes, was clear to me from beginning to end as an organic process of the unfolding of a musical idea and of Bartok's searching for a kind of perfection of the musical idea with which he started. Certainly we know enough about great music to know that composers are working with musical ideas from beginning to end that can't be described in verbal terms. This Bartok quartet—in one organic process—was searching for a kind of perfection which could be described in quite precise scientific musicological terms. And I perceived that it was not something illusory at the time of listening, because it is still with me. I bring it back to my workaday reality and I know that quartet. It belongs to me now in a way that it did not before.

Further, the bardic spans of Dylan Thomas's poems became graspable to me. In order, the words of this poem, from beginning to end, Dylan Thomas's *long spans of poetic conceit and so on became apprehensible and compre-hensible to me.*

That's actually the main thing I'd like to describe. The whole question of my subjective reactions to the various pieces is something else. I was amused at poor Schoenberg struggling so hard. A great creative artist, some of the poets, describe this experience, Goethe, Wadsworth, Blake, Dylan Thomas, all over the place they describe this kind of intense creative reality that they are in when they create.

But I've been interested to know what happened to a musician—what kind of insights he had. And this happened to me too—that I was interested and saw somehow as a reality. Beethoven's having been somewhere that Schoen-berg didn't quite make. Primarily I wanted to stress, though, this increase in the span of attention far beyond anything I've ever experienced before.

P.R., a secretary and music student

Everything became alive and beautiful. Brilliant colors, shimmering golds and greens, blazing purples and reds sparkled everywhere. The beauty and truth of one object would have been enough to keep me fascinated and awed for a lifetime. The whole world was magnificent. While enjoying these visionary delights I was plagued with terrible headaches. The right side of my head in particular felt as if it would explode twice. But I survived. I felt hot flushes on the right side of my face, the way I do in therapy when I'm confronted with something horrible.

Most of all, I felt very friendly and enjoyed the company more than any other time. Smiling like an idiot, I had a fine time; the only thing I objected to was me. It seemed as if I were a very little girl. When I got home even my mother was beautiful and she didn't annoy me at all (fantastic!). It was hard sleeping that night. LSD made me very high and gave me a sense of freedom I never felt before. This experience had a great effect on my voice. I haven't sung so freely with all 3^1/$_2$ octaves in over two years. All constrictions of the throat disappeared and I enjoyed singing tremendously. I still sound good. This proves that my troubles with singing are purely psychological.

It just confirmed my feelings that it's not the world that is so horrible but my feelings about it. I am much less angry—I have a great deal more control over it and I can put it aside. My depression lifted, and afterwards I could sing again full voice.

THE ENCHANTED LOOM

Janiger reflected at length about the powerful creative faculty that oper-ates in most of us. The comments that follow are his response to this rich database. Throughout his career Janiger thought a good deal about the powerful creative faculty that operates in most of us. In 1989 he and the author collaborated on a synthesis of his observations and Hertel's 1971 analysis of the volunteers' artwork. Many of the comments that follow are drawn from that work. Janiger believed that inspiration is a special mode of thought with a special quality over which we ordinar-ily have little conscious control, but the creative state of consciousness can be voluntarily approached and, some say, the door to it opened at will. However, we cannot quantify the creative feeling or the visionary experience. It has a quality of surprise, of wonder, of revelation, of pris-tine perceptual innocence, as if one is seeing something with brand new eyes. A term best used here is strangeness.

Poets and writers and philosophers, from the author of Ecclesiastes to Wordsworth and Henry Miller, deal again and again with the sensa-tion of awe, inspiration, wonder, and pure aesthetic delight that accom-panies a really fresh and intrinsic perception of an object, a relationship, or a state of affairs. The aesthetic experience occurs always concomitant with the feeling of something strange, unusual, or incredible. The nature of sculpture, paintings, poetry, or any artistic product is essentially an expression of this estrangement from the usual, from the stereotyped. In the case of the child, who is yet to be fully socialized, his concepts are new, groping, idiosyncratic in the extreme—strange and quite wonder-ful. Strangeness is experienced by the psychotic because of his cleavage from consensual reality.

The creative adult embraces experiences of strangeness and wonder as a gift of new sight. Often these experiences are characterized by a rising flood of afferent impulses that reintegrate phalanxes of old mem-ories, generating hosts of collateral associations and novel recombina-tions of known material. Artists, then, are those creative people who can not only experience the revelations of the aesthetic experience, but also craft them into tangible gifts for themselves and/or others.

As many scholars have noted, creative and psychotic processes have something in common. In the Jungian approach, one is not afraid of the unconscious process, but rather like Orpheus descending, the creative person delves deeply into the psyche and returns richer for the experience. Perhaps the artist is the designated person to keep those channels between consciousness and the site of creativity open, to be the warrior at the gates. In psychology, there is an area of psychopathology—depersonalization—that sheds light here. People suffering from depersonalization have a permeable membrane between their consciousness and their unconscious. They are not "crazy," but the world often looks very different to them than to other people. Such individuals do have a curtain between these layers, but at times the boundary is quite permeable and frightening, while at other times its permeability is extremely gratifying. Good imaginative writers must live close to this state of being, and James Joyce's writings portray it very well. Artists are the purveyors of all kinds of new, rich, and unusual experiences. Some people have this gift—but it comes at a price: they feel like they're observers, not participants on a stage, experiencing what we can call the "Alice in Wonderland syndrome."

In some manner, the LSD process also wrenches people loose from their well-established conceptual moorings and sets them adrift in strange, exotic, and fantastically improbable waters. As previous chapters have demonstrated, mind-manifesting chemical agents function in the minds of both artists and ordinary people in the following ways set out by Janiger:

- They provide a rapidity of thought that accelerates creative thought processes.
- They provide a basic emotional excitement and sense of significance.
- They widen consciousness to include both broad cosmic ideas and yet sharpen perception to see significance in the tiniest details.
- They provide greater accessibility to past experiences and buried memories.
- They cause things to appear to compose themselves into natural harmony.

- They intensify colors so that everything appears brilliantly illuminated from within.
- They cause the association of unrelated objects to be perceived as genuinely novel (as opposed to being without aesthetic value).
- They free the individual from preconceptions.
- They fuse the individual with the object perceived—a phenomenon that Picasso says is the most important feature of looking at things creatively. When you paint an apple, you should *be* an apple.

Whether or not one concludes from these generalizations that the LSD experience mirrors the creative process, one may certainly say that the LSD experience is innovative. One looks at things from a different perspective, employing another state of consciousness outside conventional frames of reference. Later on one can employ these novel permutations to gain greater access to one's memory banks. The result is like an explosion in a museum—all sorts of artifacts flood at you with a richness. Perhaps these substances dissolve our habitual ways of thinking, feeling, and behaving. Under normal circumstances the exquisite complexity of the mind is fairly rigorously programmed, or habituated, to keep it from breaking through into another totally chaotic reality which the Freudians call the id. Thus the mind functions much like a straight jacket, presenting us with an illusory world of unalterable reality and employing extensive fail-safe mechanisms to enable us to function within homeostatic limits. Under the influence of LSD, the habituation pattern of the brain is overwhelmed by the marvelous trains of light. There is, of course, the danger of becoming totally immersed in one's inner life, becoming almost schizophrenic. People can be utterly submerged in their internal experiences, leaving them only a grasping contact with external reality. Janiger, however, believed that one had to stretch the mind even though insanity may beckon in the shadows.

On the other hand, Janiger did not believe that LSD is a creativity tool or that it unlocks creativity. It simply makes accessible parts of the individual not normally available. People who are already artists or craftsmen when they take LSD may indeed benefit from it. If they are not sufficiently creative to begin with, LSD will not suddenly make them so.

That is, it will not by itself make a Michelangelo out of a person. It simply opens the gates to the Huxleyian doors of perception. We need to reiterate the phrase "LSD favors the prepared mind," as it is an important concept to keep in sight. People suffering from "the clod factor" never got anywhere.

Furthermore, while Janiger believed that LSD could be a powerful instrument to free the artist from ordinary perceptual ruts, he concluded that it had little effect on the development of technique. According to him LSD did not produce a tangible alteration in the way a painter paints; it did not turn a poor painter into a good painter, or a good painter into a great one. Instead, it altered the way the artists appraise the world. It made some change in their consciousness in terms of their overall understanding of their painting. It allowed the artist stuck at an obligatory level of perception to plunge into areas that previously afforded him only limited access. Nevertheless, the contrast between artists' "before" and "after" works is striking. The "before" renderings of the colorful kachina were often realistic, predictable, and drawn to scale. But the LSD-inspired drawings were more abstract, symbolic, brighter, more emotional and aesthetically adventuresome, and non-representational, and they tended to use all available space on the canvas.

Analysis of the artwork and narrative reports produced by artists in Janiger's study reveals much about LSD's short- and long-term effects on their work, that is, on their art itself. Such analysis also invites speculation into the composition of the mind. Janiger suggested that there may be in altered states of consciousness the seeds or conceptual frameworks of the different artistic styles. Can we say, perhaps, that the brain carries the germs of the so-called schools of art, that these schools did not come about randomly, but are reflections of some internal configurations of the mind? The consistent stylistic shifts demonstrated by the artists in Janiger's study may suggest that when the mind breaks free of its habitual perceptual patterns it tends to utilize alternate perceptual patterns that can be artistically expressed. For example, under the influence of LSD an impressionistic painter produced a starkly cubist rendering, a cubist produced an abstract painting, and most of the representational artists shifted toward expressionism. The liberating action of the LSD allowed the artist to recompose obligatory reality—interestingly, they did so in a recognizable set of shapes and energetic forms. LSD may be a means of opening all the possibilities, a connecting rod to specific schools of art in the sense that LSD exposes the mind to possibilities already there. The mind may be so constituted that even the variations have a certain regularity about them, a "shaping spirit," as Coleridge once called it, that is not arbitrary. Grof also believes that research into psychedelic effects reveals the psyche's structure (1994).

Janiger's study also has much to say about the creative process and the source of inspiration necessary to produce art. Specifically, the study asked whether creativity is something that individuals can uncover or turn on at will. As the excerpted reports in the previous section demonstrate, almost all of Janiger's artists stressed the ease with which details were perceived in all their particulars, an unprecedented fluidity of color, and the novelty of their perceptions. Many people reported the facility for part-whole combinations in which part elements condition the whole, vice versa, or both. They felt an inchoate but palpable conviction of creative power, which frequently enabled them to locate their strange and eerie feeling of beauty in their own heads, rather than by way of the input through their sensory receptors. This is the definition of nonobjective art; that there is an ideal vision in the mind separate from sensory perceptions.

The artists also experienced a wealth of associations, which flowed before their sensorium like a cascading Niagara, whether or not it was fed by physical stimuli from outside. In some instances these associations presented the individual with such a wide diversity of perceptual choices as to stagger and paralyze the will. Any chance remark might trigger the line along which perception is organized, or the preexisting mood, or set, or the directly antecedent stimulus—whatever was once acting as the rudder that guided the perceptual organizer. A given suggestion might provide the frame or vessel within which the subject instantly molded his perceptual cascade. If nothing else, the narrative reports show us the artists' increased awareness of alternate perceptual forms.

Many of the artists reported synesthesia in which the senses are flooded, mix together, and cross over. Sounds, for example, seemed to be colors. Elements were recombined in a new way. Thus LSD moves in the same direction that the imagination does, by springing connections that may be latent but that are not normally noticed.

Despite LSD's obvious deconditioning effect, the artists also wrote that LSD nonetheless gave them the ability to see order in chaos. It allowed them to synthesize—to see novel combinations and permutations of things. Moreover, it gave them a sense of great significance, excitement, and a deep desire to discover and invent. It fired them up with contagious enthusiasm so that they were moved to weave their vision of truth for people who had never perceived it.

In short, the majority of artists reported that they had found a way to tap their creative energies. They discovered new parts of their sensory apparatus and thinking abilities. They were able to pull things out of their memory banks and see things in their environment that they hadn't seen before. They were able to experience awe, encounter the numinous, and refashion the usual into original form. All of these are aspects of the creative process.

In the 1986 art exhibit in Santa Monica, California, called "The Enchanted Loom: LSD and Creativity," twenty-five artists commented on their work. Most notably, all were uniformly positive about the effect LSD had had on their artistic lives. They were all very taken by seeing their work again. Almost all of them expressed how much they had thought about the experience over the years, and many believed it had influenced their work from that point on. They said that if the experience wasn't the most important in their artistic development, it was *one* of the most important. None had a negative statement to make, yet only three of the returnees had chosen to take LSD again. Unlike the religious mystic who may continue to seek enlightenment continually after such an initial experience, the heightened memory for the LSD experience appears not to fade away with time nor does it follow a standard forgetting curve. Creative individuals may not need additional experiences. Or as we will see in chapter 7, the unpredictability of the LSD experience and the somatic discomforts and overwhelming emotions may take too much of a toll, deterring repeat performances.

Janiger believed that LSD alters seemingly unalterable reality. Although most of us seem to believe that reality is absolute, no matter if one is skydiving, underwater, or in weightlessness, in fact this is not so. Rather, reality may depend on our level of consciousness. Every night when we close our eyes and go to sleep, we alter our personal subjective reality. Yet from childhood on we are shepherded toward certain patterns of perception, expression, and behavior that may later actually imprison us. It is the very essence of the artist's activity is to break loose from that tyranny of structure. In this experiment LSD offered artists an additional tool to use to explore the greater depth of what they might be seeking and return to us, inspired and inspiring, tapestries in hand.

6

LSD AND SPIRITUALITY

GIVEN THE PARTICULAR EFFORT Janiger made to avoid any religious prompts in his study setting, he was surprised to find that some 24 percent of his LSD volunteers nonetheless experienced a mystical or spiritual encounter. In the pages to follow we will look in some detail at these people, whose prior interests seem to have facilitated unitive or transcendental experiences and suggest some similarities between the volunteers' reports of these experiences under LSD and descriptions of otherwise-induced mystical experiences. In chapter 7 we expand our discussion to incorporate cross-cultural uses of psychedelic plants to access spiritual realities and to provide religious and therapeutic experiences for individuals. We conclude that chapter by comparing the experiences of indigenous people and Janiger's volunteers, noting both similarities and differences.

Before we turn to the volunteers' self-reports, a few definitions are once again in order. For the purposes of this chapter, we use the terms *mystical* experience and *spiritual* experience interchangeably to refer to any person's direct, subjective communion with a deity, spirit, or ultimate reality. As theologian Evelyn Underhill defined mysticism, "It is not a philosophy . . . it is the name of that organic process which involves the perfect consummation of the Love of God, the achievement here and now of the immortal heritage of man. . . . [I]t is the art of establishing his conscious elation with the Absolute" (1974). *Religious* experiences imply similar communion, but also connote observance of personal or institutionalized beliefs or practices within what the historians of religion call *ecclesia,* or formal organized religion. Contemporary writers of the psychology of religion characterize both mystical and religious experiences in terms such as *unity,* which is the direct perception of connectedness or oneness. Thus in mystical states there is a complete lack of differentiation between the self and the object of awe and reverence, and boundaries dissolve. Opposites such as good and evil, justice and injustice, and god and humanity disappear, and all things tend toward a unified, undifferentiated oneness. Additionally, such experiences often include the transcendence of time and space and a sense of sacredness, which may present emotions ranging from awe (fascination, wonder, or terror) to a deeply felt positive mood. Profound insights can occur and are described by religious practitioners as epiphanies, theophanies, moments of illumination, and states of grace. Often people experience both understanding and redemption. Sometimes enduring changes in a person's emotional well-being, beliefs, values, and behaviors occur.

A combination of the criteria delineated by the well-known authors Evelyn Underhill, William James, Walter Stace, and Walter Pahnke (Doblin 1991) are pertinent here in providing us with a list of criteria for mystical experiences:

1. Sense of unity
2. Transcendence of time and space
3. Sense of sacredness
4. Sense of objective reality
5. Deeply felt positive mood
6. Ineffability
7. Transience

Anthropologists often make a distinction between mysticism, which they see as an individual's firsthand, direct encounter with deities or spirits, and religious experiences that are mediated through a church, temple, or some type of formal ecclesiastic structure. The ecclesiastic commitment can provoke radical reorientations and moral obligations to live a religious life (insofar as that means dedicating one's life to one's principles). By the same token, mystical experiences may provoke such when they occur within the context of a formal religious organization, but certainly need not have that proviso. Moreover, as Anthony Wallace, an anthropologist, points out (1966), religious behavior universally makes efforts to induce an ecstatic spiritual state by crudely and directly manipulating physiological processes. These include drugs as well as sensory deprivation, mortification of the flesh by pain, sleeplessness and fatigue, and deprivation of food, water, or air. As early as 1959 Wallace argued that the use of LSD and other psychedelic drugs lay in what he called a folk interpretation based on the basic psychophysiological reaction to the drug, so that the ecstatic experience is phrased for the individual as communication with the divinity. Wallace argues convincingly that the physiological manipulation of the human body, by any means available, to produce euphoria, dissociation, or hallucination is one of the nearly universal characteristics of religion. The ecstatic experience is a goal of religious effort, and whatever means are found to help the communicant reach it will be employed!

While scholars have identified many different types of religious experiences, the key elements and essential categories of *universal* religious behavior as defined by Wallace include the following:

1. Prayer: addressing the supernatural
2. Music, dancing, singing, and playing instruments
3. Physiological exercise: the physical manipulation of psychological states including the use of drugs, sensory deprivation, mortification of the flesh by pain, sleeplessness and fatigue, deprivation of food, water, or air
4. Exhortation: addressing another human being, particularly a representative of divinity
5. Reciting the code: mythology, morality, and other aspects of the belief system,
6. Simulation: imitating things in ritual explicitly oriented toward the control of supernatural beings

7. Touching things believed to contain supernatural power, such as laying on of hands in religious healing
8. Taboo: not touching sacred objects, refraining from certain behaviors
9. Feasts: a sacred meal, or eating or drinking materials that contain a supernatural force or power
10. Sacrifice: immolation, offerings, and fees
11. Congregation: processions, meetings and convocations
12. Inspiration: a temporary union with a god or spirit
13. Symbolism: manufacture and use of symbolic objects that may represent the divinities themselves

For many, the sense of unity or awe is one of the most arresting aspects of a mystical-religious experience, as Wallace points out in his discussion of the physical manipulation of psychological states. The concept of an absolute unitary state of being as one in which all perception of multiplicity of being is eradicated has been nicely delineated by the anthropologist Eugene D'Aquili and his colleagues. In this state individuals directly apprehend absolute unity with themselves, others, and the universe. Subject and object merge and boundaries to the self are weakened. Reality itself is perceived as oneness. Attached to this experience is a profound and intrinsic sense of underlying beauty and goodness. That is, the universe is perceived as whole, good, and purposeful. When people leave this state, they do not perceive it as having been an illusion, hallucination, or delusion. Rather, they see it as the fundamental reality that underlies all reality.

It is important to note that this sense of reality differs enormously from that traditionally validated by scientists. Psychologist Charles Tart makes a distinction between baseline states of consciousness (b-SoC) and discrete altered states of consciousness (d-ASoC). He argues convincingly that rational consciousness is merely one type of consciousness, equally valid with that induced spiritually, or one, for that matter, induced by LSD. Science arises from our rational, baseline state of consciousness that perceives reality as an amalgam of multiple discrete beings in emotionally neutral subject-object relationships.

This deer kachina doll was the subject used by all of the artists participating in Janiger's study. All but one of the artists' pieces reproduced in this section are interpretations of this object. (The last piece is an artist's self-portrait.)

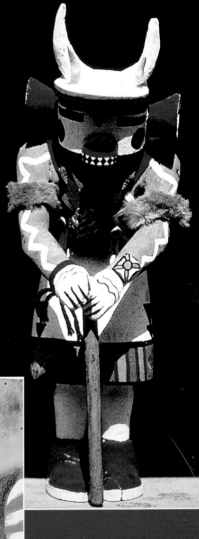

Painting of the kachina doll produced under the influence of LSD.

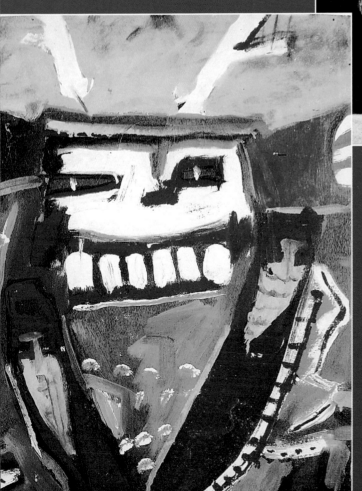

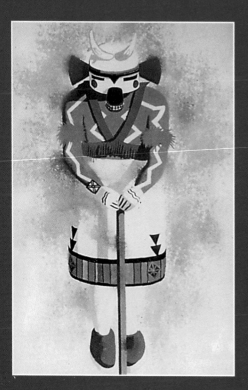

An artist's first rendition of the deer kachina doll, produced prior to ingesting LSD

The same artist's rendering of the doll while under the influence of LSD. This pair of drawings appeared on the invitation to the exhibition of art produced in Janiger's study.

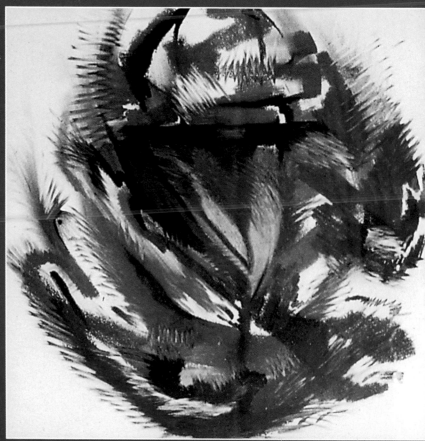

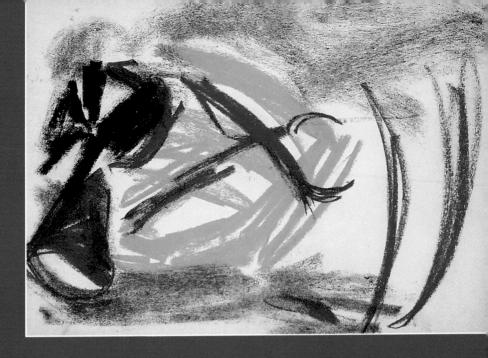

Drawing produced before ingesting LSD

Drawing produced under the influence of LSD.

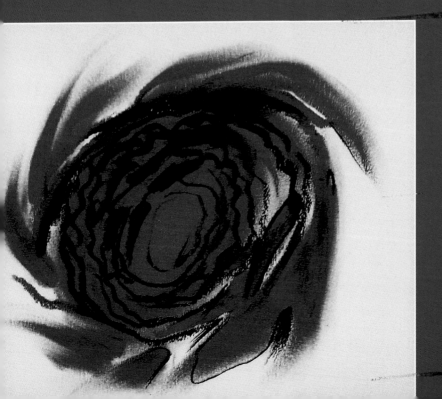

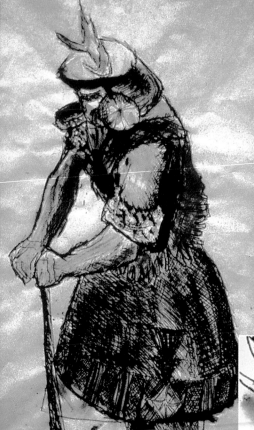

Drawing produced before ingesting LSD

Painting produced by the same artist under the influence of LSD.

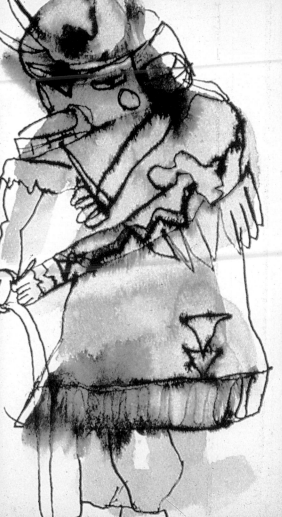

Painting produced before ingesting LSD.

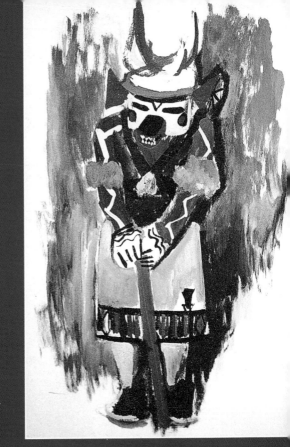

Painting produced by the same artist under the influence of LSD.

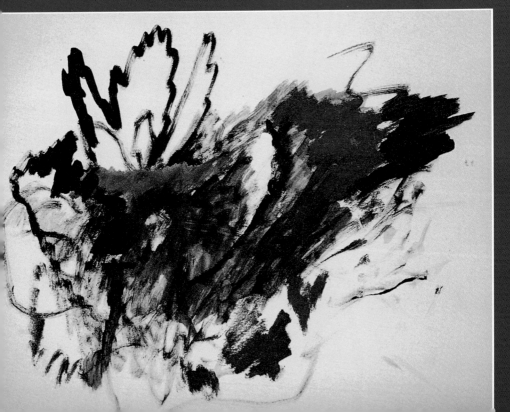

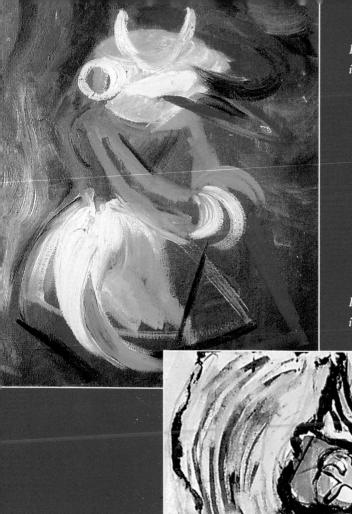

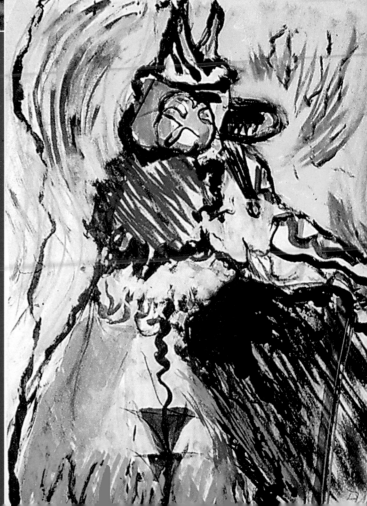

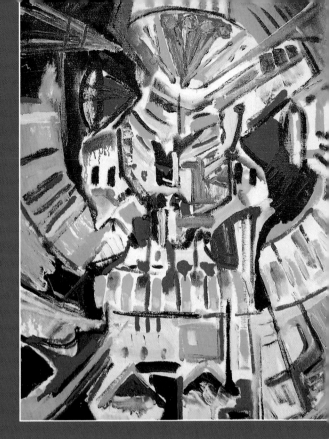

Painting produced under the influence of LSD.

Drawing produced under the influence of LSD.

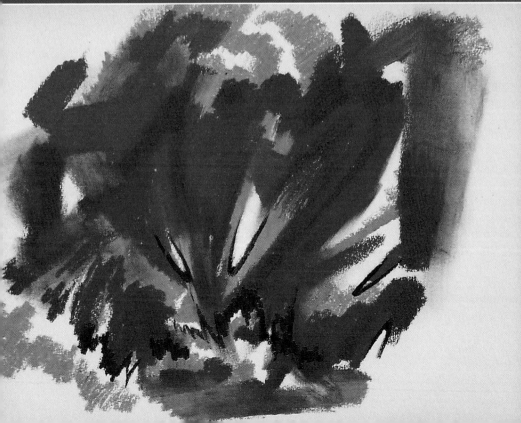

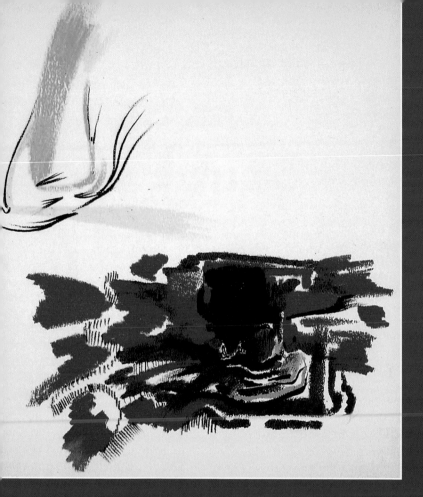

Painting produced under the influence of LSD.

The first two images in this triptych are the artist's self-portraits created before ingesting LSD; the last image was produced under the influence of LSD.

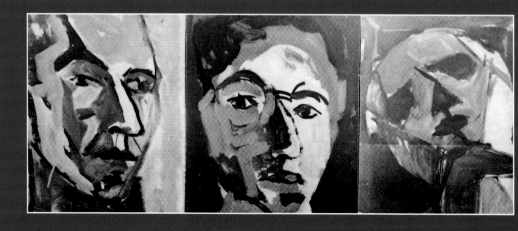

The absolute unitary state, on the other hand, arises from discrete altered states of consciousness. The absolute unity of being can be considered an ultimate trance state. For D'Aquili and Newberg, the trance stage progressively becomes intense, with a blurring of the boundaries of individuals until they perceive no spatial or temporal boundaries at all and experience absolute unity, devoid of content. The self-other construct is obliterated. Ultimately, the person experiences a movement from a baseline orientation in external reality to a more intense sense of unity with the rest of the world and an increasing loss of a sense of self and other. The person now can lose individuality and experience a sense of absorption into the object of focus or the universe in general. As D'Aquili and Newberg argue, a person reaching the absolute unity of being not only becomes one with that object and experiences a breakdown of the self-other dichotomy, but also "the object that he is absorbed into is also broken down, which gives rise to an experience of unity with all things."

After the unitary state is experienced it is most often interpreted as the presence of the Absolute or union with God. In a Buddhist context it is seen as a void. D'Aquili points out that a common result of this experience is freedom from fear of death. In large groups this freedom can be adaptive to survival if at least some members of the group experience it and bring that message back to the social group at large, allaying anxiety and fear. D'Aquili also argues that an emotionally integrative consciousness exists side by side with our rational and analytic selves. This has implications for both scientific objectivity and religious intuition. He suggests that during mystical experiences the right hemisphere of the brain produces a rush of emotion that powerfully validates the perception of unity without being subject to left-hemispheric analytic process that distorts the original message.

As rare and individualized as these experiences are, those who have them universally interpret them as being absolutely transcendent, or in some sense ultimate or beyond ordinary experience. They are remarkable—and worth investigating—for their revelations not only about the nature of human consciousness, but also about the nature of reality.

STUDIES OF MYSTICAL EXPERIENCES

Long dismissed by science as a realm fit only for theologians and philosophers, the study of mystical-religious experiences has only recently moved to a foremost position in the research agendas of many scientists. Today discussions of mysticism not only include the voices of religious scholars and philosophers, who have long validated the mystical experience, but also psychologists, anthropologists, and neurobiologists, many of whom increasingly argue that human psyches, cultures, and brains are wired for spirituality.

In the early 1900s two works set the stage for science's entry onto the scene: philosopher (and later psychologist) William James' *The Varieties of Religious Experience* (1961) and theologian Evelyn Underhill's *Mysticism: A Study in the Nature and Development of Man's Spiritual Consciousness* (1974). Working from primary accounts, both books systematically analyzed mystical experiences, generated definable categories and lists of criteria such as those presented earlier in this chapter, and challenged prevailing opinion that mysticism equals pathology. James lucidly argued that our normal waking consciousness—Tart's baseline state of consciousness—is only one of many alternate consciousnesses available to us, each equally valid and appropriate for different applications. This basic concept cued the development of the psychology of religion and consciousness research.

Structural anthropology in the first half of the century furthered this work by describing and validating the diversity of cultural patterns of kinship, myths, and rituals. In so doing, anthropologists challenged Western science's xenocentric assumptions of normalcy as belonging only to Western society. Over time, anthropologists became "adamant that what is normal is defined within the context of the particular society" (Benedict 1934). Further, as anthropologists such as Anthony Wallace (1966) and cross-cultural religious scholars such as Walter Stace (1987) began systematically describing the mystical rituals of indigenous people, it became clear that the core mystical experience described earlier by historians and theologians pertains, as well, across cultures. In the end scientists were left with no option but to take mysticism seriously as a normal, if relatively infrequent, component of human experience, at least in postindustrial society.

Acknowledging the persistence of this core experience, psychologists became increasingly serious in their research into spiritual consciousness. Some, like David Wulff and Michael Thalbourne, seek to discover psychological profiles that enable some people to experience spiritual epiphanies more readily than others. Others, like Charles Tart (1969) and Stanislav Grof (1994), have challenged the simplicity of Freud's tripartite model of the human psyche by developing new models of consciousness based in part on conclusions from their research into spiritual consciousness.

Anthropology and psychology have also intersected in the study of the role of psychoactive substances in inducing transcendental and unitive encounters. As we will see in chapter 7, anthropologists such as de Rios (1984) have shown that psychoactive plants have been valued for thousands of years in many cultures for their ability to facilitate mystical/transcendent experiences in ritual contexts. Religious scholars like Huston Smith suggest that these mystical experiences have provided the bedrock phenomenological foundation for most of the world's religions (2000). Additionally, since William James' experiments with nitrous oxide, some psychologists have argued that, under appropriate conditions, psychoactive substances can occasion profound mystical experiences that are indistinguishable in description and impact from naturally-occurring mystical experiences that result from prayer, fasting, solitude, or other practiced austerities.

In 1961 Harvard doctoral candidate Walter Pahnke conducted the famous Good Friday experiment at Boston University's Marsh Chapel. In this study Pahnke and his academic advisor, Timothy Leary, then at Harvard, sought to test two hypotheses: 1) that psilocybin could facilitate mystical experiences in volunteers with religious orientations and in a religious setting and 2) that such experiences would result in persisting positive changes in attitudes and behaviors. Pertinently, Pahnke did *not* seek to prove that psilocybin produces mystical experiences regardless of context or volunteers' predisposition. Indeed, Pahnke gave psilocybin capsules to ten white, male divinity student volunteers and active placebos to another ten students before a Good Friday service. Using an eight-category typology of mystical experience drawn from Stace and three methods (an interview and two sets of questionnaires) of quantifying the volunteers' experiences, Pahnke proved his first hypothesis to his own satisfaction: that psilocybin could facilitate mystical experiences in prepared volunteers "indistinguishable from mystical experiences described in cross-cultural literature." A six-month follow-up to the study seemed to more than prove the second: The students who received psilocybin experienced more persisting changes in attitudes and behaviors, including basic vocational changes, than did the control group. A twenty-five year follow-up conducted by Rick Doblin generally supported these conclusions (1991). In fact, the relationship between psychoactive substances and authentic mystical experience has become so well accepted by its advocates that they suggest replacing the culturally-laden terms *psychedelic, hallucinogenic,* and *psychoactive* with the more precise *entheogenic,* meaning "to become divine within" (Ott 1995).

However, other research presents us with problems about the seemingly simple relationship between psychoactive substances and mystical experiences. In 1972 theologian R. C. Zaehner criticized the Good Friday conclusions, citing flawed questionnaires and a failure to distinguish among levels of religious experience. He refuted Pahnke's first claim that drug experiences can be authentically religious, arguing that while drugs can produce two types of mysticism (the soul merging with nature and the soul merging with an impersonal absolute), they cannot produce what he called theistic mysticism in which the soul "confronts the living, personal God." Doblin's follow-up study also qualified Pahnke's unconditionally positive report by revealing that Pahnke significantly underemphasized the psychological struggles his psilocybin volunteers experienced and failed to report that thorazine was administered to one student who later described his experience as a "psychotic episode."

Other research—ironically, Leary's Concord Prison study—has challenged Pahnke's conclusion that psilocybin induces enduring positive change. Between 1961 and 1963 Leary sought to prove that "the consciousness-expanding properties of psilocybin would provide prisoners with insights into their own criminal behavior and could therefore be used to change future behaviors." Thirty-two Concord inmates volunteered for six-week programs during which they received significant preparation, between two and five doses of psilocybin, therapy, and post-release support. However, while Leary hypothesized that psilocybin would reduce criminal behavior as measured by recidivism rates, a follow-up concluded that the "long-term recidivism rate was no better than the average base rate for recidivism for inmates at Concord Prison" (Doblin and Forcier 1998). Huston Smith foreshadowed Doblin's reservations when he wrote in 1964, "Drugs appear able to induce religious experiences; it is less evident that they can produce religious lives" (93), if by religious life one means dedicating oneself to enacting one's values on a daily basis.

Most recently, psychologists are joining with neuroscientists to investigate the relationships between consciousness and reality. Rudimentary technology in the 1950s and 1960s was sufficient to reveal differences between the brain waves of people in baseline states of consciousness and people deep in meditation, but it could not explain why the waves changed or what regions of the brain were being activated. Recent developments in brain-imaging technology, however, allow scientists to be much more precise, and the last fifteen years have seen the rise of an entirely new field known as neurotheology that investigates the neurobiology of spirituality and religion. Leading proponents in this field argue that the compelling commonalities among mystical experiences across time, cultures, and faiths suggest—if nothing else—a common neurobiology or structure and function of the human brain.

Working with Eugene D'Aquili, radiologist Andrew Newberg has used X-ray technology to map the brain activity of Tibetan Buddhists and Franciscan nuns during moments of peak spiritual experience. The researchers found that both deep meditation and intensely spiritual moments of prayer produced definable patterns of neural activity in the regions of the brain that govern attention, emotions, and our sense of orientation in time and space. Taken together, these patterns can account for the characteristics of mystical experiences: oneness, transcendence, objectivity, sacredness, positive mood, ineffability, and timelessness (2001). Corroborated by the work of other researchers (see Austin 1998 and McKinney 1994), these findings suggest the human brain is hardwired to experience what D'Aquili and his colleagues have been calling "the absolute unity of being" as an objective reality.

Some neuroscientists argue that mystical phenomena are completely caused and contained by functions of the brain and the mind. Others argue that mystical reality, the presence of the divine, exists "out there" in the external world and can be experienced by human beings through the mind and the brain. Newberg and his coauthors refuse to take sides, contenting themselves instead with identifying eight different areas of the brain that can be understood either as creating spiritual or mystical states or as allowing the individual to access these states under certain conditions: meditation, sensory deprivation or overload, LSD ingestion, and so forth.

Obviously, powerful hallucinogens like LSD affect the operation of the brain. However, the current ban on human LSD research prohibits a direct comparison between the brain activity—as pictured by brain images—of people during spontaneous mystical experiences and LSD-induced spiritual experiences. We do know that LSD stimulates the hippocampus, thus producing changes in both the hippocampus and amygdala, which are associated with generating vivid or hyperlucid (extremely vivid) hallucinations. Three areas of the brain—the amygdala, the hippocampus, and the neocortex in the temporal lobe—are involved in the production of these vivid hallucinatory experiences. These very structures are involved in visionary mystical experiences, within an extremely complex web of neural structures and their interconnections (see Austin 2001, Winkelman 2000). We can also infer from descriptions of LSD experiences, such as those in Janiger's study, that it can affect the same brain regions activated in Newberg's images, but we won't be certain without further research.

JANIGER'S SECULAR RESEARCH MODEL

Unlike Pahnke's deliberate use of seminary students in a religious context in the Good Friday experiment, Janiger strenuously avoided providing any religious or mystical prompts for his volunteers. Both researchers thus adhered to the general rule that any drug's effect depends on three factors: the properties of the drug itself, the setting in which it is taken, and the "set" (psychological makeup) of the people who take it. Pahnke sought to prove that psilocybin could induce spiritual experiences in people with a religious set in a religious setting. Janiger sought to discover a core LSD experience by using a broad spectrum of volunteers in a secular and naturalistic setting.

Specifically, Janiger devised as neutral a setting as possible. To eliminate a religious context that would be expected to influence the volunteers' experiences, Janiger made sure that there were no rituals present. Religious music was not played as a matter of course although about half of the volunteers chose to accompany their experiences with music they either brought with them or chose from a large selection of records at the research site. More generally, and as chapter 2 details, Janiger tried to eliminate distractions, and whenever possible friends, lovers, and spouses were asked not to come to the sessions. As few external stimuli as possible were permitted. Seeking to avoid another extreme, Janiger also warded against the type of white-coat laboratory neutrality that he believed to have negatively affected other research results by keeping the Wilton Place house surroundings plain, ordinary, and natural. Some people ate; others not at all. Volunteers were always free to leave the house to go to a nearby coffee shop or spend time in the Wilton Place garden if accompanied by a staff member.

Naturally, Janiger also refrained from influencing the volunteers' mindsets other than to reassure them that they would grow from the experience and that the experiment could be stopped at any point. The volunteers were not told what kinds of experiences to expect, and most had no prior experience with psychedelics. In a few instances some individuals were given LSD on two or even three separate occasions. Moreover, Janiger deliberately recruited the most average and "normal" cross-section of the population that he could to reduce the possibility that a common set would undermine his search for LSD's core characteristics. It should be noted, however, that all the volunteers were either Americans or foreigners who had been living in the United States for some time. Janiger also thought it prudent to accept only those volunteers who demonstrated sufficiently strong egos so that LSD's disorienting properties would not make them panic. Thus he asked candidates such questions as whether they had ever gone to Carlsbad Caverns, how they had enjoyed the stalagmites and stalactites, and what they thought about space exploration. People who responded positively were considered to be anchored firmly in their own concepts of themselves and at small risk for negative LSD effects.

Given his attention to the secular setting, his care to avoid influencing his volunteers' mind-sets, and his preexisting belief that LSD does not inherently produce mystical experiences, Janiger could not have predicted that 24 percent of his volunteers' reports would resonate so closely with classic descriptions of spiritual transcendence. Let's turn now to a sampling of personal accounts from those volunteers who did.

VOLUNTEERS' EXPERIENCES

As we read volunteers' narratives of their mystical experiences, we note the occasional fractured grammar and syntax. Many volunteers wrote these lines at the end of the day on which they were given the LSD, while others provided their comments on the thirty-day follow-up questionnaire that Janiger sent to them.

I.P., a musician

In a report written five weeks later after LSD ingestion, this musician reported his effects six to seven hours into the experience. He had entered a "New Dimension of Meaning."

I mean these last words to be taken in an absolutely literal way. Entering this New Dimension can be compared only to the reaction of a man, blind from birth, who suddenly gains his sight and for the first time, experiences color. Five weeks later, of course, the danger exists—and I take what precautions I can against it—of superimposing onto this experience a layer of rational thought. While thought can help to organize the mass of raw material one has accumulated, there is a risk that this very rationality, coming from a lower, more ordinary part of our awareness, may reduce the experience to what can be understood from an ordinary state, discolor what one has seen with all the old conditioning and opinionation [sic] and thus debase the essential quality of the New Dimension to which one has been granted admission.

The LSD produced in me an essentially religious experience. None of the conventional symbols or verbal accouterments of religious practice, with one notable exception, were in evidence. But the essence of religious experience, as I had always imagined it, permeated the afternoon to a degree of intensity that I had never known, except for brief, fleeting moments in the past.

These remembered moments from long ago, however, occurred mostly while I was composing. They had been so intense and special that there was no mistaking their absolute similarity to the far more prolonged LSD state. It was for me a kind of reassuring evidence. Without this basis for comparison, I might be tempted not to trust the LSD-induced ecstasy, or at least to be much more suspicious of a state of exaltation of such fantastic proportions which had come about through no inner efforts of my own.

Finally about thirty minutes after taking LSD, I began to notice that a little Indian doll on the table across the room was vibrating in a strange aura of light, as though it were trying to come to life. . . . I began to notice soft but inexorable barriers taking form in my mind, blocking out past and future. Only this eternal Now [h]as import, only this moment counts. Strangely static and unlike the constantly traveling present—moment of the ordinary state matters to me, seduces me, rivets my attention. Attention on what? On nothing, just on the Now.

I.P. began to listen to music, and had this response.

It bores me, it gets in the way. One and a half hours later and still nothing more remarkable than a strange, eerie prelude. Disappointed. Restless and disconsolate. Lethargic and heavy.

Gradually, he realizes that the experience has started to become different.

No, I have. I have grown extremely sensitive. My flesh is charged with emotional responsiveness to the Mozart E-flat symphony. My skin seems microscopically thick and porous so as to admit the music more easily. The inner lines of counterpoint are suddenly so clear. The dissonances are so penetrating, and the bass-line is positively alive. It jumps and strides with a kind of cosmic purpose. I am very sensitive but my real emotions still have not been engaged. My mind is racing, speculating. I have no visual phenomena.

What is beginning is the extraordinary flowing or remaining sensation that pervades the next hours, a feeling that my entire being is partaking of or taking part in an event of ultimate importance. It is as though my body were being carried along in an increasingly powerful flood of energy and radiance. My listening is extraordinarily acute. My emotions are very near the surface, always available. What emotions? I can't say. The outer frame remains passive and delicately balanced to allow what is inside to be actively to receive, actively to perceive, actively to be. There was much resistance. Great waves of negation came and went. Inner talking from the rational center. A kind of lone man holding down the mental fort while everyone else is out in force for the incredible goings-on elsewhere. That person in me is talking, talking about the fact that he simply cannot evaluate what is happening. That he's not sure this is at all pleasant, but is, in fact pretty suspect. That this is the cheapest kind of mental side-show provided by the Mephistophelian medicine-man and his little blue pills which are producing this psychically phenomenal slight-of-mind performance, this phony circus of sensations and hallucinations, monstrously parading under the name of spiritual experience; that somehow a state of mystical ecstasy should have a sense of dignity, of exaltation, and inner quiet, not this raging river of special effects.

As the day progressed, the resistance became weaker and finally disappeared. In the blaze of light, at the height of the experience, I lost valuable time in moralizing, rationalizing and making agonized attempts to 'see' myself in this unfamiliar state from a seat high up in the amphitheater of my mind. The intensity and radiance of the journey kept growing. I had no company except an occasional momentary visit from Dr. J., so this part of the afternoon (three and a half hours into the trip)—Shattering intensity of feeling. Filling every second was the flowing, the endless, flowing sea of energy which streamed and roared and pulsed through my entire being. Then of course, there was the music. Mozart, Bizet Symphony, Moussorsky Pictures, the suite from Strauss's Der Rosenkavalier and my own incident music.

My reaction to these pieces began with the conventional response but gradually took on a new character. It was as though the remaining ecstasy that flowed through me has washed away my patience with the exterior posturing of music. I felt that I saw directly into its heart and was interested only in what the music was really saying, remaining totally indifferent to how it was dressed.

The feelings were so intense and were so much from this New Dimension of feeling that there is very little I can say except to report them. Their intensity was almost unbearable, their nature unknown and indescribable. They seemed to have to do with a kind of love we cannot experience as we are. For a few moments I understood them and would recognize them as Truth. Now

I can only remember that I understood for a moment. The understanding is gone, with only the memory of it remaining.

While my innards were being ripped apart by the intensity of these feelings, while I was streaking like a rocket through this emotional world, I recalled Gilbran's words about Sorrow, which carves us out inside so that we may contain more joy. This was precisely what I felt in those hours. I regretted not being in the country. I resented the enclosing room and ran out into the little courtyard. The tree, which I looked at from the doorstep a few moments later, affected me perhaps more deeply than anything that day. It said everything. It represented everything. It was God's bounty. It was Beauty, it was Fertility, it was Providence, it was divine Grace. I actually could not bear the intensity of the feeling and had to come inside. My body was now a torrential river, streaming and flowing. At the same time it felt like some unknown stringed instrument being played by an unseen hand, which drew its bow across me to release a kind of music for which there are no words. Totally indescribable.

Somehow the significance of things, from ash trays to symphonies, to trees became the primary object of perception. I saw not a table but quite clearly and simple tableness [sic], the reality behind the object which at this moment had far more concreteness than the table itself, the nature of table. This all came to me in emotional terms, or in terms which I have no adjectives to describe, except that these terms expressed meaning beyond words or concepts. In this connection, there was much impatience with the man-made and deep craving for the creations of nature.

The visual hallucinations were one of the more entertaining features of the afternoon. There is no denying the extraordinary splendor of what I saw. The room trembled with violets and bluey reds, shimmering and radiating from pictures and objects. I could not for a time distinguish between sight and sound. Later Mozart's melodic line was filling the room at that moment. I couldn't at that time distinguish between sight and sound. Later woodwind harmonies released ethereal glowing purples and pinks in shafts of radiant light which streamed out from a picture in precise synchronization with the music.

I felt that moment of incredible exaltation. Filled with this realization: I am, in this very instant, free. I am free from every petty negative emotion. I am devoid of anger, of jealousy, of fear. I suddenly saw that I did not need these absurd encumbrances. I suddenly felt what it might feel like to be a man. I exulted. I laughed.

It was an unbelievable, a totally unexpected journey. One has been there and back, but the nature of the traveling of the destination remains a haunting enigma. One is galvanized into attention, attention to a fantastic adventure which shatters, sears and exalts one's entire being and yet which one cannot depict with even one really true word.

Even after this all too brief voyage, however, it becomes clear to me that this new dimension and the nature of its reality is somehow related to Man's reason for existing on the earth; and that any life lived without a constant inner need to "be" in relation to this dimension is a life without meaning.

Z.G.

A five-fold banquet of the soul. The yellow paper I have brought with me to write is dancing, bending, shedding an unearthly radiance and bending the point of the pen so that my script is shaky, wilder, larger than usual and the lines short and running down the side of the page. Writing under LSD is like trying to write during an earthquake while standing under a cascade of ice, mint, lavender, and orange. The body shakes and only an effort of the will provides the impetus to jot down the vacuous notes prompted by unleashed immensities. The five senses have taken off in different directions and are bringing back reports of their wonderful discoveries.

I was aware of the terrible limitations of the mind. . . . Feelings of unsurpassed love and beauty come and go like warm waves of wind. The snow of a forest melts into a singling river and dark, mercurial feelings of compassion press down the bell sound of monsters into the fur-lined echoes of an ocean.

One doesn't discover the self because there is no self. One only discovers the self under LSD, that is, one discovers oneself in the pose dictated by the specifics of LSD and through its wild intoxicating tropical glamour and fantasy through its unbridled gushing all including, all combining merger of thought, idea and sensation in a collage of super collages; Matisse, oranges and lavenders, Parisian tones and Vienna depths of blue and ice.

LSD overthrows the normal thought process based upon sensory perception where if one sense is involved in an experience of importance, unusual, painful or pleasurable, it obtains or commands the attention of the brain while the other senses sink into the background or more truthfully perhaps, attempt to cooperate in providing additional information on the experience at hand. Under the influence of LSD, a sense of sight seems to be driven inwardly into its own storehouse of experience and undergoes a forced regurgitation of images, colors and textures at the same time that it distorts whatever visual stimuli it is willing to receive from the outside. The imagination, fired by a new freedom and basing itself mostly on the heightened sense of sight, turns into a vision of Dionysian proportions. The entire body leaps into a paroxysm of aesthetic pleasure. Unimaginable dimensions are added to the sense of hearing and to the psychological implications inherent in music. One's being seems to be driven by a maelstrom of succeeding delights into uncontrollable laughter and joy. Joy comes swelling up in tremendous waves that rack the entire body and become frightening in their intensity. The omnipotence of the living moment triumphs in a total manner over the gray residue of death floating in the memory. Consciousness is not a flowering in or within a universe but universe itself flowering and no barriers, no limitations. Joy arrives like an inevitable visitor, the psychological result of power and power is felt within the tenement of bone and racked flesh as the harmonious result of a surprised will flooded by the imagination.

C.V., a minister

At 11:00 A.M., until past 1:00 P.M., I had feelings of unutterable emotional pain which swept through me in wave after wave, coming out in moans, groans and sobbing with the words, "no, no, no, no" issuing forth. The analogy came to me and I said it aloud, that it was as though all the feelings that ever had been in the universe had to pass through me as though I was a small funnel. It was as though all of history's emotions were still existent somewhere and in this period of a few hours they had to flow through me.

The realization of all the suffering that has been and now is a part of the world seemed to flood into me, and I felt with shattering intensity all the different kinds of hurt of men, women and children everywhere.

The thought came bursting forth that "This is what God has had to go through" standing by, loving mankind, while mankind goes on hurting himself and each other through all his ignorance and injustice. I said aloud repeatedly, "Poor, poor, God. What God has had to go through." The thought came flooding in that this is what the cross means . . . the standing by, only able to offer love to man and to suffer for him till he experiences that love in a way that lets him stop hurting himself and his fellow man. This is what the cross means, I said: "now I know what the cross means. If we only knew, we wouldn't go on doing this to each other. How does God let us go on existing?"

It didn't seem to be that I was hurting, but just that I was being a vessel through which hurt was being expressed. I felt no need for pity or sympathy as a particular person. I was just an expression of mankind's hurt. Every conceivable kind of emotional pain was flowing through a funnel, and I just happened to be that funnel.

After quite some time of this, the realization came to me that in all this welter of emotion, I had not experienced the emotion of anger or hate. This seemed strange to me, that in the uncontrollable experience of all sorts of feeling I was feeling no anger, and I asked myself, "where was the hate," and I tried to dig up the feeling of hate, but I could not. As I searched for it, I became finally convinced that there wasn't any to find, and I said aloud: There isn't any hate, I can't find any hate. I couldn't understand it but I was convinced of the truth of it, for I had no ability to repress anything. Later that day, I made some sense out of it.

The volunteer had no hallucinations; nothing changed in the least. The entire experience was completely emotional in nature. He had no feelings of self-rejection. He experienced himself as just another poor human creature doing his best to find his way through life.

We seem to feel in life that to be totally overwhelmed by emotional hurt is to be lost and destroyed. This is not so. Hurt is not destructive. It is the refusal to bear hurt that is destructive, making us act against others, blaming them, punishing them, and engaging in self destructive defenses.

In retrospect, if the person is willing to accept the LSD experience of any hell which may lie within him, then fine, let him go ahead and my blessing goes with him. I feel the LSD experience was a very growth-producing experience but we must choose to experience suffering as a free oral agent [sic], not be pushed to it by another.

In this account, we see an individual's spiritual journey within a religious context of belonging to a doctrinal church, rather than an individualistic experience by itself.

S.W.

The overriding feeling of the LSD experience was one of wholeness, unity and a kind of unutterable joy and contentment. Everything that I saw was incomparably beautiful, soft and serene. The colors were all soothing pastels, greens, flesh tints—they were exquisitely soft. The visions were infinite. At one time, I watched a fountain and gradually became the fountain itself, or rather—I became the actual flow of the water. It was an extraordinarily joyous experience. Several times I felt disembodied. This was strongest when I was watching monastery steps appear. I seemed to float two or three inches above myself.

I had a feeling of wholeness and completeness that I have only seen described in the experience of mystics undergoing illumination. The feeling of oneness with the entire world seems to me the most essential and dominant part of my feelings. It was persistent and clings to me now, several days later.

I felt completely submerged in the energy that made up whatever visions I saw. In a sense this was a kind of immunity that brought great happiness. I lost all sense of myself as being something independent and I became part of the universe. I looked into the mirror and kept seeing faces I did not care for. The first was a rather cruel, hard, conquistador type; next a foppish boulevardier. Next, a thin-mouthed lawyer. Face after face appeared in the mirror and I tore them all off like masks; none of them I liked. I worried about not being able to go back through the mirror. I would turn it over to God. With this thought, I had a vision of what appeared to be a mixture of a cradle and an altar, with a stream of light shining down, which I took to be God's blessing. The vision was short lived.

In this report, we see the transitory nature of the mystical experience; nonetheless it had an effect on the individual that may have lasted for most of his life. The very nature of the mystical experience is the persistence with which the memory of it remains active.

P.Y.

Everything was shattering. Glass, etc. I seemed to see out as though I were at the rear of a stage and there were five or six curtains, recessed. Backstage of each was a separate compartment of the mind. Traveled down through caverns, some beautiful but mostly hideous with lizards and more lizards. Lizards coming out of each other from the navel and more and more and more.

I tried to pray but it would lighten up a little and then get gray again. I became small and smaller. Until there wasn't anything except what I thought was the ego left and finally that disappeared into the bare ground and I was nothing.

She described a second LSD trip as follows.

First, I went over vast, vast, vast regions of desert with absolutely no sign of life. Then I began the upward journey into the light. I entered the light. A white light, not yellow like fire, or lamplight or sunlight. As I entered more and more it seemed to pin me, penetrate me, through every cell. I was aware of it entering every part of me. This feeling of being surrounded and penetrated by Light lasted what appeared to be a long, wonderfully long time. I was perfectly relaxed in body, and I felt indescribable joy, something even much stronger. I became one with the light. I was the Light. I saw the most intricate beautiful meshing of what we might describe as gears in geometric designs so complex and complicated that I was amazed and awed. I merged with these workings and became them. Then, I was in an unearthly world of more and more and more pure, pure beauty. The colors and forms were again unknown, the beauty excruciating. The intensity of the experience faded.

My conclusions: a tremendous awe and respect and a great sense of well being, a nothing-can-ever-matter-too-much-again feeling after having experienced and seen what I believe to be the workings of the Cosmos. I do not wish to seem conceited but I believe that a part of me was transported to the Godhead. An intense realization of the importance of Order and Beauty. In the I Am state, there is no such thing as love, hate, duty obligation, etc. I can no longer think of God in the old way, as Our Father, but instead it must be Very God of Very God, or Light of Lights.

P.C.

My hands felt enormously sensitized. It seemed as if with my hands, I could hear resonances—feel the vibrating beat and pulsation of them. The basic resonances. The C-Majors of the universe. There seemed to be this magnetic pulsating beat. Just to be one with it, to commune with it, to be part of it—the beats, the pulsations—for one afternoon. This was where new doors opened where new fields lay fresh and green and sweet. This was the thing to experience. People never intruded in my experience.

Some of those gardens in front of the houses were beautiful beyond description. The beautiful blending of the colors of rose and grass, of willow-grays and flaming scarlets, of buff yellows and deep purples. I took a blossom of scarlet thistledown. . . . It was revelationary [sic]. To look at the individual tendrils of that beautiful delicate blossom and to see the richness and the fulfillment that was there. Each one of those delicate tendrils shoots out in a tremendously livid scarlet color and then is capped by a beautiful crown of gold.

Things seemed to move around me in different planes but with one focal point—one source for everything. A focal point that was itself was not in focus [sic]. Past-present-future. I was one with all these at the same time. I was timeless. It was a Peter Pan sort of feeling. The whole experience was childish and psychotic. It was completely without self-consciousness, completely without vanity, completely without self pity, completely without desire. . . . When I say, these words childish and psychotic, I mean them in almost a holy way. For during this experience, for the first time in my life, I was able to contemplate without concentration. I'll get back to the religious part of this experience a little later. The physical act of writing was very difficult at this time. My hands had this extraordinary sensation of sensitivity. My fingers wanted to spread out, splay footed, like the foot of a frog. When I wrote, the ink from the pen didn't seem to want to stay on the paper.

I seemed to be able to see things as total pictures rather than in the piece-meal way that we so often look at something. I was like in a childhood psychosis. I was completely amoral in the most literal sense. I felt that I was "in" on causes, one with causing forces but was no part of them myself. I was a beast in a completely objective, non-pejorative way. I had no insight because I was in. And I wondered: Is this God? A beast with no insight.

I was undergoing a kind of half-human, half-animal experience. The problems of the conscience did not bother me at all and moralisms became very superficial things. I thought of moralisms, and anti-moralisms and anti-moralism-moralisms. God was the Creator, the Force, but he too was completely amoral. He was neither a God of Love nor a God of Hate. A God of Compassion or a God of Wrath. He was simply the Being at the Center, the *beast with no Insight. The question that disturbs me in this view is: where is evolution, where is our progress? It seemed to me that Life was just a spinning thing, orbiting around a nuclear God who created it, who held it together with the force of his gravity, but who did not influence it. It seemed as if Evolution had backed up against itself and that there was no Evolution at all. Doesn't evolution influence morality and morality evolution? Isn't evolution the real basis for morality? This experience was completely amoral.*

A.E.

The bewildering aspect of the experience with LSD for me, lies in the fact that the Infinite actually is presented to a human mind incapable of grasping the spherical concept of the Infinite. As a result, the human in this experience actually feels himself caught up and immersed in the experience. The infinite whirls before the bedazzled mental gaze of the humankind, reducing him to stunned and awed incomprehension. And this incomprehension is at the same time being bombarded by a veritable star shower of comprehension.

Through the action of LSD, the human mind has been separated from its limited restrictive and destructive world of angles and hard facets and has been brought face to face with the Reality of the Infinite. Every measurable angularity of the world he has constructed is knocked out from under man in this experience and he finds himself inundated in immensity.

A day later the volunteer recorded further insights.

I return from this experience, humbled even as I am exalted and inspired. The humility and the exaltation become one as I perceive that in order to encompass the Infinite, I must be absorbed by the Infinite. Yet, even as I realize this, I also realize that it is not a case of losing my identity in the absorption. Rather I now know that in my absorption in the Infinite I find my identity of individuality for the first time. For in being absorbed, I have expanded to comprehend.

In this experience, I was keenly aware of fragmentation. I attempt now to diagnose the sense and meaning of that fragmentation. For instance there was a demand for a drink of water by some sense yet I was not aware of actual thirst. Hands and feet moved in certain necessary motions yet seemed to be moving of their own volition. In fact, I was conscious of faint surprise at the precisions of movement of a member such as a hand, so completely frag-

mented were my coordinates and sense of being in command of the member.

Throughout the experience I was clearly and keenly conscious of my conscious mind being poised in a position of command. At this point my basic spiritual desires deemed to be directing the mind in the meaning of the phenomenon. I was both undergoing and observing. Thus, I was able to comprehend the fragmentation that was taking place.

As I recall the experience step by step, I realize that it was the unnatural rigidity of angularity that was being fragmented. The human sense of angles, faces of immeasurable dimensions was utterly shattered. Thus, mentally, I caught a glimpse of the glories of the Infinite. Moreover, these glimpses were never disturbing. Rather, I was conscious that in this fragmentation, I was observing Reality for the first time. Also I was keenly conscious of the self-command that I must emerge from the experience retaining the spiritual meaning of that which I had glimpsed.

In the beginning was the Word and the Word was with God and the Word was God. God is the Infinite, Infinite Love, Infinite Order and Intelligence, Infinite Wisdom. Yet even as I touch on these attributes of God, the Father, I see them as One. Only my human concepts could be fragmented. Throughout the experience, the Logos, or Word which is One, grew in coherence even as it expanded in beauty, order, and glory. As I came out of the experience all truth was contained in the immeasurable concept of the Logos, or Word.

F.D.

This woman's hope was that LSD would release some latent creative talent in her.

About an hour after taking LSD and just before I fell asleep at night, I had a brief interlude of pleasurable sexual awareness. Another friend, Claire, was present. When we were sitting silently side by side, I had a feeling completely pure and true because it came solely from within me of perfect communication with her. I was really tuned in on her wavelength. I could sense her moods and feelings. It was not communication of minds, but wordless, very real touching of spirits. I was not aware of myself except as pure spirit in a new realm of pure spirit. I felt somewhat superior to the others in the group preoccupied with visual or auditory sensations still tied down to the everyday world. My world of pure spirit, colorless, soundless, tasteless—seemed a step closer to the Eternal Truth? God? The feeling was quite definitely non-denominationally religious and profound. I don't mean the feeling of superiority but the translation of myself into spirit only.

I entered into an enchanted garden. I was like a child needing guidance and the next thing I knew, I was a child crossing a rainbow colored bridge and I was in an enchanted garden. There were tall trees and a dark pond with water lilies all looking quite natural but I knew that it was a Russian fairytale garden. There were no animals and no other people. I was in and out of this garden during the whole first half of the day. I was just there and this state of being gave me the most wonderful feelings of peace, innocence and truth. When Oz [Janiger] came up to me and asked me how I was feeling, I answered curtly, fine. At that moment I knew perfectly well who he was, who I was, where I was and what was going on. I was annoyed, though, for being called out of my garden to answer questions. I wanted to speak Russian instead of English.

At one time when I returned briefly to my garden, the branches of the trees I was looking at danced a ballet to the music coming from the other room. The green of the pine needles suddenly broke up into all the primary colors and the clouds formed modern designs in the sky. The feeling of communication with others would become all engulfing for a moment. I was fully aware of every day reality while still feeling the effects of the LSD.

What was the overall meaning of this experience for me? It confirmed what I knew, suspected and hoped for about myself. The garden proved to me that I have succeeded in working out my own philosophy of life and I am now at peace with myself. The memory of that real profound peace I found in the garden will give me added strength now—for reaching deeper into myself than I ever have before. I found a rock there, solid enough to build my whole life on. LSD opens new doors or enlarges the horizons of my perception and in my case, stretches the span of emotional perception starting from a new depth within me and reaching out to a distant world of pure spirit.

K.Q.

This volunteer, a musician, went to a park with the monitor about an hour after ingesting LSD. His report is summarized due to its length.

He felt detached from himself and from his surroundings. He felt a oneness with nature. He was struck by shapes and colors of incredible intensity and he had an ecstatic physical feeling of surrender that was almost overpowering. It lasted most of the day.

He reported that he had feelings that he must have felt as an infant, a sort of *déjà vu*. He then had a series of paranoic suspicions of the doctor, including the thought that he was a storm trooper who carried a gun. The doctor was his keeper but he did not have negative emotions of hatred or destructive impulses. He was imbued with an overpowering sense of love for all things and an intense yearning for love, protection, and acceptance. He saw Bosch-type images of an anal, visceral, and bloody nature. Later, in the park again, he had an almost completely unrealistic sense of detachment from this world. Then he went to the beach. The ocean was an incredible sight. He could see for miles. He noticed the detailed markings of birds in flight from afar. He was aware of the slow rhythm of the ocean's ebb and flow and conscious of some large pulsation of the earth. He felt himself to be part of them.

S.Z.

The first thing I noticed was a diminishing of self-consciousness and cessation of inhibitions. After a while, my hearing increased to incredible acuteness. I heard the air-compressor in the air-conditioning machine. The proper study of mankind is man. So, on our walk, I spoke to the gargoyles which twisted on a baroque column, and discussed the leaf situation with a caterpillar, and worshipped at the spray of rainbows in a lawn sprinkler and said hello to a red flower breathing on a pulsating undulating white wall. I had lost my personality and felt: "What a good riddance." For two hours, I received and knew and soared and laughed, but it was not that novel in protoplasm, not me. It was someone, nice and fine and good and completely benevolent, someone who accepted the world. I saw my friend, Jane, as a great artist, a sculptor whose hands could create the heavens and earth as a Michelangelo or Rodin. I dove into the shining swimming pool of her bright green and infinitely clear eyes, and was immediately tangled in the sunlight, the daylight in her mind.

What determines what you see under LSD? I offer this analogy. We are walking up a spiral staircase inside a round stone tower. On each floor there is a window. In the basement there are no windows, there we see panic, paranoia, devils; on the first floor we see out a little slit of a window; we see the bright lights; the wonderful taste of the electric field of that saline solution called a Kosher Dill pickle. We are sensual. We hear mockingbirds sing like a feathered choir of angels. We see the sidewalks glitter with stones of fire. We see the animistic world living, breathing, walls inhaling, oil paintings with living skin moving with muscles under the surface; we know what Heraclitous [sic] meant; Pan is alive. We close our eyes and we see fireworks, skyrockets opening with a sigh and dropping flowers of fire lighting up the night.

But this is only the first floor. We walk up another flight and on the second story, the window is wider and we see that fiery self which is seeing, translating, composing. And this self, with the glory of God shining round about it, is a far more gripping sight than the jewels of fire, the living breathing flowers, the visions of delight, the sound of laughter in the corridors of space; for this self is the interior lightning which flashes and thunders with the power of a vast demi-urge, broadcasting an electro-magnetic field of force which can control, command, summon up these visions and spirits from the vast deep, play with them a moment and let them fall. What else can we do with this force?

Psychotherapy? Yes. Exploration? Yes. An expedition, which goes out to climb Mt. Everest and fails, is a failure. But an expedition, which goes out to find what it can find—serendipity, or anything interesting—cannot fail. We don't know where we are. We are probably in the same position with LSD as Francis Bacon was with electricity. He took a needle and rubbed it with amber, and Lo! Bits of salt jumped upon the needle and clung to it. That's all he could do with electricity. We can't do much with LSD until we commission expeditions to go out and bring back whatever they find with no preconception about what they should find. We should recognize that the higher a man has climbed in the round stone tower, the wider the window he will find. His findings may have little in common, if he is on the tenth floor, with the person on the first floor who is having a ball with baubles and dill pickles.

We may discover the common-sense world of things, and individual consciousness while it actually exists, is the world seen from the most narrow window on the lowest floor. The emergent evolution of man's consciousness requires that we widen the window. LSD, the Mexican Mushrooms, the Yogic meditations, are means to widen the window. Then we may find that the common sense world and our separate personalized way of looking at it are a part of what Einstein calls the Fourth Dimensional Space-Time Continuum, a part of what the mystics call the Divine Ground. Here in this Universal Sea, in which separateness does not exist, we may find true meaning and ecstasy.

We may discover that we may reach this Universal Sea, this Continuum, this divine energy—not by verbalizing, not by Aristotelian syllogisms, but by direct contact, direct experience, in which we allow it, by acceptance, to flow in us, to beat in our veins—and more, that we not only compose and create this undifferentiated sea into form, shape, color, sound, but we limit it also by using it for small purposes. As we climb up in the tower of our minds and see out from wider windows we may discover that the thing seen and the person seeing are manifestations of that same divine energy. We may then find that good may be defined as union, while evil may be defined as separation. To lose our personalities in a higher form of energy is like a bird's molting his baby feathers to learn to fly. The individual personality is a means of separation, a means of reducing the universal sea down to separate things, a means of cutting ourselves off from the flow of energy that is always in us; LSD breaks down those walls of separation and liberates the deeper selves which can only come out and function in a mind striving for unity—rather than for defenses against unity.

The layers on layers of individual selves may be likened to Salome's seven veils. As we tear off the surface personality we can let the deeper individual self begin to live, and sensually experience the world as it is meant to be experienced, intensely and ecstatically. As we tear off the veil of that individual self, we can feel that we lose the need for sharp identity. At this point, we can go in two directions, toward more personal power as some of the Hatha Yogas have done, first by showing that their individual will can conquer all manner of physical obstacles. Or, we can go in the direction of identifying ourselves with all the divine energy that flows in that universal sea. This seems to be the way LSD points.

We may find by continuing down this road that man has one purpose: to find his eternal self, the spark of God that flames in him, to realize that this spark is made of undifferentiated flame from the universal sea; to see the purpose as rejoining this flame with all flame as a tributary, caused by snow melting, caused by condensation of sea water in the clouds, rejoining the sea. Is LSD a mystical experience?

The volunteer at this point in his narrative examines six denominators that all mystical experiences share. Unfortunately, we cannot guess the source, if any, of the list he presents.

- *Pioneers into the unknown must either be struck dumb by ineffable wonders—or must invent new terms which are unfamiliar to those left behind.*
- *The world is suffused with dazzling splendor, illuminated as if from within.*
- *The world is suffused with significant meaning. Nothing is insignificant. Everywhere you look is wonder. And the meaning means something intensely good.*
- *There is a feeling of nowness. There is no past and no future. This moment, this ecstasy, this awareness is all-important. Happiness is not something to be experienced sometimes in the future, on the weekend, on vacation, after retirement. It is now. And you would not change a thing.*
- *There is a feeling of warmth, goodness, love, benevolence—but not in the solemn sense—in the sense of fun—of laughter, great grinning at everything, as if your personality were the Cheshire cat and everything about it had disappeared except this uncontainable smile. It is loving, as the sun shines, inevitably, inexorably and with infinite fun.*
- *There is a feeling of continuum, of flow, as if we were as individuals, no more than whirlpools in a river—but whirlpools with wills, and we can will that two whirlpools can come together and join as one, or that we disappear and join the river. Once you feel the continuum flowing in you, you are no longer troubled with yourself for you know it isn't separated from anything else.*
- *There is an ability to distinguish between the real and the unimportant. And all things, which are symbols of the real—as a car is a symbol of power—a mink [coat] is a symbol of love—these become unimportant. That which is immediate, intense, ecstatic and satisfying, is real; that which is indirect, symbolic, postponed, tending toward separateness, is unimportant.*

We can play with our minds, the dance of creation and destruction—we can build real castles in our minds and destroy them—we learn that the creative force of the universe is continually playing, continually creating, like the wave-forms in the oscilloscopes and cathode rays. And our minds are of this creative force, for as it makes spiral nebulae and supernovas, we can make wave-forms with our minds, without any instrument except our liberated wills. And this play is more important to the human race than most work; for it is the kind of scientific play which through inadvertency or serendipity discovers the richest and most fruitful hypotheses.

We can love without being loved in return. We can love for the pleasure of loving as flowers give off odor. We do not need to get "our way" nor do we need to be hurt. For we are a part of the living, breathing, undulating, bright shining God and we see him not only in the pulsating wall of granite, in the wave-forms of the dancing wood-grain, but we see him in ourselves, in the fire behind our eyes, the flame on our foreheads—and we feel this glow like a shooting geyser in us, and we call it love. To turn it off, because it is not returned, would be to castrate our minds, and constipate the flow of this fire— it must flow—for it is our means of having life and having it more abundantly.

E.R.

A Hindu religious monk, E.R. meditated for four days before ingesting the LSD, sleeping only a little bit. A psychic picture unrolled before his mind, symbolically providing a clear procedure as to how the LSD experience can be embarked upon as a religious journey, from a religious point of view. This process presented itself in the form of a revelation, which worked exceedingly well as he put it into operation, and produced the following evaluation of his experience. It is interesting that he did not really describe his experience, but rather presented an intellectual model.

The human body is like a flowering plant. The stalk of the plant is the spine. The brain, which resides at the top of the stalk is the bud of the flower which is capable of blooming. The folds of the brain tissue are not unlike the folds of a rose bud. The pineal and pituitary glands are like the pistal [sic] and stamin [sic] of a flower. But the human plant could be more likened to the century plant which blossoms only once in its lifetime. The reason why our brain does not blossom as it should is that we do not live natural lives. The human race has imposed all sorts of abnormal impositions on itself, both physical and mental. The proper growth and function of the brain is not allowed to take place. Prior to this revelation I had assumed that oriental religious terminology such as "the thousand petaled Lotus residing in the center of the head" was merely poetic symbology for psychological effects. This new concept translates the idea into organic chemistry and gives us tangible substance with which to deal. The flights of mind, the spiritual and psychic rebirth of the mystic can be had permanently if the flower of the brain can be made to blossom.

This flowering or activation of the glands of the brain is brought about by what might be called life force, for want of a better term. The Hindus use the term Prana. This life force is being produced and collected in the body at all times and we cannot exist without it. The key to this life-force are the sexual organs which lie at the base of the spine and might be likened to the roots of the stalk of the plant, where our spiritual nourishment has its origin. The purpose is to draw this life force up to the glands of the brain rather than let it be expended through emissions of the sexual organs. This is not easy to do.

Z.I.

LSD as a spiritual releasing agent produced much the same experience I previously underwent during intense yoga practices and meditation in the Himalayas of India. There is no doubt that LSD affects a person in the same way as meditation in its advanced stages. But LSD does not seem to leave permanent after-effects. One must return to the normal state of his mind or to the advanced state of mind if he is already established in it. However LSD can be useful as a spiritual agent. It encourages one to try to explore more in the higher regions of consciousness and to experience more inner power or even experience self-awareness for temporary periods. It gives a shifting or variety of experiences rather than one true pointed establishment.

Before using LSD, a person should have a strong nervous system. A weak nervous system may receive a bad reaction. A man should have some power at least of emotional retention. Secondly it should be used only for those who wish to better themselves and not for those who want to use these powers for degeneration.

The ancient Vedas of the Hindus have mentioned three basic ways to mys-

tical experience: I) meditation (higher), 2) yoga practices (middle), 3) herbs or medicine (lower).

VIEW FROM THE SPIRAL STAIRCASE

As noted earlier, Janiger strongly believed that there is nothing inherent in LSD to cause a spiritual experience. Rather, he believed that it is simply the social engineering in particular societies that gives rise to spiritual expectations from psychedelic substances. By extension, he believed there to be nothing inherently spiritual about the LSD experience, and he carefully refrained from providing a spiritual context in his research. He often indicated that he considered the relatively high incidence of spiritual experiences among the volunteers to be an anomaly in the data, or what the psychologist Schumaker would call a corruption of reality (1995). In his book Schumaker argues that religion can be an expression of the unique human ability to modify and regulate reality in ways that serve the individual and society. Nevertheless, 223 of Janiger's volunteers reported spiritual responses that fit classical typologies of mystical experience such as those discussed earlier.

As the above excerpts illustrate, some of the volunteers clearly experienced a form of D'Aquili's absolute unity of being. Whether they meshed in perfect synchronicity with the geometry of the universe, "pulsed with the C Major" of it, described themselves as absorbed into the infinite or "transported to the Godhead," their narratives testify to an apprehension of direct unity with the universe in which the self's identity is lost, fragmented perceptions cohere, and opposites (such as love and hate) disappear. Notable here is the repeated description of this "I Am" state—and of the volunteers themselves—as completely benevolent, characterized by "unsurpassed love" and the absence of anger or negativity. A conspicuous exception to this trend is P.C.'s description of I Am as absolutely amoral, but even this report communicates the volunteer's deeply felt positive mood.

Just as convincingly, the volunteers relate experiences of transcendence and sacredness as objective reality. In many instances, they felt themselves rise beyond their usual realm of understanding into a "new dimension," what one report calls the Eternal Now, where time is meaningless. For many, this transcendent plane was shot through with a sense of sacredness or the presence of God. These volunteers felt themselves in the hands of God, "penetrated by Light," at "a five-fold banquet of the soul," exalted, serene, and one with "the One." The narratives also convey the message that the sacred, transcendent, and unitive state is a reality underlying or existing alongside our normal perception of reality, one that may, perhaps, be glimpsed only briefly and without hope of accurate description, but one that nonetheless sears those who glimpse it so intensely that they cannot forget it and are to some degree transformed.

To the extent, then, that we compare the volunteers' experiences to historical descriptions of mystical experiences not induced by drugs, it is not difficult to conclude that LSD can indeed provoke mystical ecstasy. Perhaps, as William James speculated of nitrous oxide, LSD can lift the "filmiest of screens" that separate our everyday consciousness from the one that has access to mystical revelation (Walsh and Vaughan 1993). Perhaps, reflecting D'Aquili's explanation of the mystical experience, LSD stimulates the right hemisphere of the brain to incapacitate the left, thus allowing an integrative consciousness to perceive reality without mediation from our analytic selves. Perhaps, reflecting the recent discoveries in neurotheology, LSD activates and deactivates certain brain-center operators, resulting in the sense that boundaries between the self and surroundings have dissolved, time has ceased, and reality is both endless and interwoven. Even our sense of objective reality has been traced to a specific region of the brain, one that may be also be activated by LSD and account for the volunteers' conviction that their mystical experiences were unquestionably real rather than delusions or hallucinations.

In light of all this evidence, the question at this point seems *not* to be, as Janiger thought, why did a full 24 percent of his volunteers report mystical experiences, but rather why did so *few* report them? We can pose several partial explanations. First, it is a truism that the effects of all psychedelic substances are dosage-dependent, including the accessing of spiritual realms. Numerous experts including Chandler and Hartmann (1960) historically delineated a psychedelic versus a psycholytic approach to the use of LSD. Osmond, in his work on LSD and alcoholism (1957) showed how high dosages of LSD caused a group of subjects to have genuine transcendental experiences that he believed were responsible for their continued sobriety compared to a control group that was not given such a dosage. Pahnke's research with psilocybin, mentioned earlier, had that goal as well: to induce a mystical experience with doses in the medium range. The data gathered by Janiger utilized what we would consider to be a low dosage of LSD. The low dosage, based on milligrams per kilogram of body weight, would not necessarily enhance the mystical experience among individuals who were not already committed to such a perception of their reality.

Second, the effects of psychedelic substances are notoriously influenced by setting and set. As chapter 7 will illustrate, in tribal societies where psychedelics are believed to be sacred and used ritually after extensive preparation, they perform reliably as tools for accessing spiritual realms. In contrast, Janiger made every effort to avoid predisposing his volunteers in any manner, trusting that the experiences of unprepared volunteers in a naturalistic setting would reveal some inherent, culturally-neutral pattern of LSD effects. Ironically, that pattern appears to have been idiosyncrasy, or distinctiveness peculiar to each individual himself or herself, fully in keeping with the cultural pattern of Western society, where individual primacy—what some psychiatrists have called the egocentric self—is ascendant. As anthropologists keep reminding us, culture cannot be ignored. What may also have occurred is that the volunteers' *lack* of preparation in fact masked LSD's spiritual effects by highlighting its psychophysiological effects, which in turn were seen through the lenses of personal life history, educational background, life experiences, and so forth.

Finally, we can speculate that cultural influences pervaded volunteers' mindsets so deeply that they failed to recognize aspects of the mystical experience. As we saw in chapter 3, a number of the volunteers displayed anxiety (and on occasion, debilitating anxiety) when they took LSD. Janiger related this anxiety to LSD's distortion of their everyday perceptions, which they did not expect. A second explanation is that the dissolution of their egos, the part of the self to which Westerners cling so tightly, literally scared the hell out of them. Rather than experiencing the melting away of the "I" as a unity experience of merging into the universe, as people in Hindu societies or contemplative traditions very well might, some in the strictly American study population experienced fear and panic. It is here that we can most clearly see the crucial role played by the prepared mind. People trained to seek the loss of self as evidence of sacred communion are likely to rejoice in an experience that eradicates multiplicity. The volunteers—prepared by their culture to value and expect baseline consciousness that perceives a rational universe dominated by discrete ego—experienced loss of ego as the sinking of a life raft in a sea of unknowns.

Thus it could be said that the fact that 24 percent of the volunteers experienced spiritual responses at low dosages and with nonconducive settings and psychologies implies more about LSD's irrepressible potential to induce mystical experience than about its limits as an entheogen.

In June 2001, at a conference held annually by the U.S. National Institute on Drug Abuse (NIDA), de Rios participated in a symposium entitled "Hallucinogens and Religion: Historical to Scientific Perspectives." As the symposium organizers pointed out, in the United States hallucinogens have been classified as Schedule I substances under the Controlled Substances Act because they were considered to have high abuse liability and to be of no therapeutic value. The focus of the symposium contributors, however, was quite opposite, as the participants argued for psychedelics' historically established spiritual role and their potential in psychotherapy.

Both the volunteer narratives in this chapter and anthropological research clearly indicate that psychedelics can occasion profound mystical experiences. Even if we do no more than accept the testimony of Janiger's volunteers or accept other research that links mystical experiences with improved health (see McCullough and Larson 2002) and freedom from fear of death (see Pahnke 1971 and D'Aquili 2001), it seems probable that psychedelics do, in fact, have therapeutic value when used deliberately. Moreover, de Rios's research on cross-cultural psychedelic plant use has documented the vital social and religious roles that LSD-like plants have had historically and, in some settings, still have today and their lack of abuse potential when they are used ritually

(1990, 2002). Several, mainly cultural, factors probably contribute to this low incidence of abuse.

First, de Rios's findings show indigenous peoples highly value psychedelic plants for their access to supernatural power and the unitive experience. Thus the substances were given in ritualized religious settings in natural environments with all the senses engaged, elders and religious leaders were present to ensure a smooth interior spiritual experience, and these were laden with educational content to reassure the individual. Moreover, people had specific expectations of what they would see—what de Rios (1984) has called "stereotypic visions," which were eagerly sought after to indicate that contact with the realm of the sacred had indeed occurred. The limited availability of botanical psychedelics may also figure into the absence of abuse. Finally, the classic psychedelics' unpredictable noneuphoric effects, such as nausea, vomiting, and diarrhea that we saw in the narratives in chapter 3, certainly reduce abuse rates. The U.S. ban grew out of uncontrolled/undirected drug use and misreported effects in the 1960s. These considerations suggest that NIDA's ban is more a consequence of cultural attitudes in the United States—where people take psychedelics without preparation or guidance—than of the properties of psychedelics themselves.

It is probably more accurate to speak of LSD's dangers than to assume its high abuse potential. The dangers are real, especially when the substance is used idiosyncratically by the unprepared. As the above excerpts demonstrate, even LSD experiences that are, on balance, extremely positive, can contain elements of paranoia or frightening visions. (Some researchers argue that the presence of psychological struggle disqualifies psychedelic peaks from the company of genuine mystical experience. See, for example, Tart and Smith 1998.) As K.Q. shows, some volunteers believed that there were people involved in plots against them. Once again Janiger ascribed the negative experience to the ego commitment of the volunteer, casting paranoia as a defense mechanism of the ego. Thus as the LSD effects began and individuals began to lose a sense of integrity and boundaries, they might experience anxiety, nausea, and vomiting. Their experience is comparable to that of a snail that crawls from its shell. At that moment, everything seems much larger than life and indeed must be frightening. In an early paper, de Rios and Katz (1971) wrote about the role of music in the psychedelic experience to provide the structure that the psychedelic removed—what they called the "jungle gym" in consciousness. In tribal drug-induced consciousness, music is the stabilizing factor that literally programs the visions that individuals have. In allowing his volunteers to choose their own music (if any) to accompany their LSD experiences, Janiger lost an excellent opportunity to measure the effects of different types of music, including spiritual effects. Of course, hindsight always shows us decisions that could have provided us with different and interesting data.

Janiger himself was very clear about the potential dangers of the LSD experience for people who lack strongly organized egos, as his attention to screening candidates indicates. Even in the midst of potential spiritual revelation, such people might suddenly panic as their sense of self dissolved and they lost their "hidden observer." Spreading out into the environment, feeling that they were not themselves, and knowing that they were not as secure or organized about themselves as when they had a certainty of the world around them, they might well respond with terror rather than reverence.

Janiger also ascribed negative responses to any volunteer's past trauma. He agreed with Freud that the mind has a conscious and a subconscious part, divided by a thin membrane. Neurotheological constructs are beginning to postulate the actual neuroanatomic and neurophysiologic mechanisms responsible for this dichotomy. In this construct the subconscious is kept at bay until something causes the membrane to become more permeable, allowing unconscious content to seep into conscious awareness. Freud, of course, focused on dreams and slips of the tongue, when the conscious aspect of the self is shut down and unconscious forces have more energy to pervade the individual's awareness. Whatever pierces that barrier releases material that ordinarily would not be accessible to the mind. For Janiger LSD was just such a substance, equally capable of lifting the veil to usher in the marvelous as to summon frightening, repressed memory. And as we see with criminals such as Charles Manson, LSD obviously will enhance already existing personality characteristics and may also increase the potential for psychosis in an already-fragile personality whose ego strength, again, is not able to withstand the loss of sense of self.

Moreover, people undergoing LSD experiences put themselves in a position of jeopardy because they simply can't be as alert to their surroundings. For example, a person walking down the street in a LSD state could easily be hit by a car while attending to interior activity. In that very real sense, LSD can deprive people of some of their capacity to deal with the world.

Are these dangers reason enough to dismiss the importance of LSD's apparent relationship with the numinous? We think not. Rather, they emphasize the crucial role that culture and preparation play in determining LSD's effects. Given a safe, ritualistic setting and people prepared to experience drastic shifts in consciousness as beneficial, much of the danger ebbs and the likelihood of mystical experience rises.

Newberg and his colleagues have placed this mysticism within an evolutionary context, indicating that a positive benefit would accrue to a population with some access to the experience of unity and of overcoming the fear of death. Like artists who travel to the creative realm and bring back to us their visions, those who experience the ineffable return bearing word that just beyond our everyday consciousness lies a reality *and a self* of undifferentiated wholeness, benevolence, and reconciliation. Word from the scientists has it that we are, in fact, and have been since the dawn of humanity, wired to experience this ecstatic state. In Janiger's study, despite all the odds, LSD proved to be a path to revelation.

We turn now to the question of psychedelics' reliability as catalysts of spiritual consciousness.

7

PSYCHEDELICS
AND CULTURE

AS WE HAVE SEEN, LSD has the surprising potential to facilitate positive, mystical experiences even in an environment that is banal and ordinary. This chapter poses the question: To what degree does culture determine the effects of LSD and LSD-like substances? Since human research with LSD has been off-limits since the mid-1960s, we are obliged to turn to anthropological reports on the use of psychedelics among indigenous peoples or within the context of protected religious institutions to see the way that other cultures have used LSD-like substances to achieve specific results.

Janiger attempted to tease out of his data a set of noncultural "core" effects of LSD, as if the cultural expectations of his volunteers could be totally discounted. However, as noted in chapter 6 and as anthropologists have been demonstrating in all fields they study, one cannot simply factor away culture. It is demonstrable in the gait with which we walk, in the language we speak, in the emotions we feel, in the food that we taste and the odors we smell, in the music we like. In fact, one could go on at great length about the effects of culture on all aspects of human behavior. With Western culture's stress on individualism, it is not surprising that Janiger sought to reveal the idiosyncratic effects of LSD on his volunteers, nor is it surprising that the data revealed a marked pattern of idiosyncrasy, in which volunteers viewed the psychophysiological effects of LSD through private lenses of their own life histories.

Not all cultures, however, have approached psychedelics with the same expectations. De Rios's and other scholars' cross-cultural research with psychedelics clearly shows that a particular set of beliefs and values concerning psychedelics will help to structure an individual's private experience. In fact, both tribal societies and religious subcultures make great use of certain characteristics of psychedelics. For example, suggestibility, which was deliberately ignored by Janiger, is widely employed to direct the psychedelic journey toward predetermined goals. Ironically, many of Janiger's volunteer self-reports mention feelings of surrender and a strong inclination to be led or directed by another, but they had no one to follow.

In this chapter we summarize the results of de Rios's anthropological field studies and compare her conclusions to Janiger's. While Janiger's Los Angeles setting may have been a pleasant one, it was much more artificial than the world of de Rios's Peruvian and Brazilian participants, and the groups did not share similar expectations of what would occur under the influence of psychedelics. Janiger's study occurred at a time in American society when individuals had few expectations about such experiences. Yet despite obvious differences in set and setting, a careful comparison of Janiger's data with de Rios's reveals a handful of psychedelic core characteristics that appear to transcend culture, as well as the undeniable importance of culture on psychedelic effects.

THE ANTHROPOLOGY OF PSYCHEDELICS

De Rios, a medical anthropologist who has specialized in studying psychedelics in a variety of cultures and throughout history, lived in the Peruvian Amazon and coastal areas in the 1960s and 1970s. As a graduate student in 1967, she studied traditional folk healers on the Peruvian coast—farmers who used a plant psychedelic called San Pedro (*Trichocereus pachanoi*) to treat psychological and emotional disorders of their neighbors and clients. From 1968 to 1969 she lived in an urban slum called Belen in the Amazon city of Iquitos, Peru, where she conducted extensive research on the use of the psychedelic vine ayahuasca by ten healers and their patients. In 1970 de Rios was a visiting scientist at the Smithsonian Institution in Washington, D.C., helping to prepare an exhibit called "Man's Use of Drugs." The data she gathered from these projects formed the basis for her book *Hallucinogens: Cross-Cultural Perspective* (1990), which examined the important role that plant psychedelics have played in human history and prehistory. Subsequently, as professor of anthropology at California State University, Fullerton, she taught a number of courses on psychedelics and culture, including one on tribal arts of societies where such substances were widely used. In the 1990s she made two visits to Brazil to study a psychedelic church, the União do Vegetal, where ayahuasca is used as a religious sacrament.

Over the years de Rios met frequently with "Oz" Janiger informally and in a variety of professional meetings and talks. She was keenly interested in learning about the LSD studies that he had conducted more than a decade before she went to live in Peru, particularly as she had been given LSD by a psychiatric colleague in Peru in 1968, when LSD was still being used in clinical psychiatric research. In 1989 at her invitation, Janiger and she prepared a paper on LSD and creativity, the results of which have been incorporated into chapter 6. It was, however, only after his death and in preparing this book that she had the opportunity to reflect more broadly on the similarities and differences that link Janiger's LSD research in Los Angeles with her own cross-cultural research on psychedelics. Most of the information yielded by her comparison did not surprise her. After all, she had always argued for cultural universals in the psychedelic experience. Human beings are members of the same species—*Homo sapiens*—and the psychedelics tend to fall into a particular chemical class. One would thus expect to find similar themes and motifs in LSD-like experiences. Yet the comparison also reveals just how influenced by culture and setting these themes can be.

Psychedelics in Human History

Throughout her studies de Rios found that psychedelics have always been viewed in human cultures as a double-edged sword. On one edge is psychedelics' perceived potential to provide access to authentic spiritual realms, and many cultures have consistently used LSD-like substances toward this end. Proponents of this position believe that changing our body chemistry or neurochemistry allows us to attain realms of being that are not ordinarily available to most men and women. Both Newberg and D'Aquili's work, discussed last chapter, and the shamanic rituals discussed below are good examples of this approach, although it should be noted that the aforementioned authors are deliberately equivocal about whether God exists outside of us or is a product of our neurochemistry. The other edge is psychedelics' perceived potential to deceive—rather than to enlighten or sanctify us. In the rational world of European/American heritage there is no spirit realm to access, so psychedelics are seen merely as tricksters of the mind. Certainly, theologians and sages historically distrusted psychedelics' capacity to induce authentic spiritual experiences. Zaehner's critique of the Good Friday experiment is a modern example of this stance, but it is also evident in the Vedic tradition, which prioritizes meditation and yoga over medicine as legitimate routes to mystical experience. One of Janiger's volunteers, I.P., expressed this point of view well during the initial phase of his LSD experience, describing it as "the cheapest kind of mental side-show provided by the Mephistophelian medicine-man and his little blue pills which are producing this psychically phenomenal slight-of-mind performance, this phony circus of sensations and hallucinations, monstrously parading under the name of spiritual experience." (See page 128.) We should perhaps note, however, that I.P. viewed this early judgment as his rational mind's stubborn resistance to what was, in the end, an authentic mystical experience.

De Rios has also studied the major roles psychedelics have played in human history and the influence of cultural evolution upon those roles. Over time societies have tended to move in the direction of greater complexity, and de Rios has investigated psychedelic use in societies of hunter-gatherers, incipient agriculturists, intensive agriculturists, and ancient city-states. In many tribal hunting-and-gathering societies, every adult man would have had at least one psychedelic experience in his lifetime, often during male initiation rituals at puberty. And in a contemporary Amazonian tribal community of eighty people, as many as twenty-five adult men might take ayahausca twice a week or more in ritual ceremonies. In small-scale societies these rituals appear to enhance group cohesion and reaffirm local cultural values and beliefs.

It is possible that psychedelic rituals developed first in such hunter-gatherer communities where human beings and animals coexisted most closely. Several contemporary tribal societies that use plant psychedelics in religious practice report that they learned about these plants from deer, reindeer, or wild boars in their environments (de Rios 1990). Despite the apparent nonadaptive potential of such animal behavior (they may be more vulnerable to prey species while intoxicated), there are more than 150 reports by scientists of animals seeking out these plants (Siegel 1989). At the very least, this data may point out the antiquity of psychedelic use in human society since hunters and gatherers were the most likely to observe animal plant use carefully and to imitate this behavior in prehistoric times.

As de Rios and David E. Smith, the founder of the Haight-Ashbury Free Clinic in San Francisco, explained in a paper they published in 1977, as societies became more complex they developed restrictive laws to limit access to drug-induced altered states of consciousness, thereby permitting fewer and fewer individuals to enter these realms. Likewise in state societies, access to psychedelic substances—and the power and knowledge they were believed to possess—was typically reserved for religious functionaries and kept from the average man or woman. In ancient civilizations where we have records of plant psychedelic use, limitation of drug access was without doubt related to two perceptions of threat. These perceptions were: 1) the supposed power of the hallucinogenic state and the "power" believed to be conferred upon the user to control or harm others through magical means or witchcraft, and 2) the potential for LSD-like experiences to undermine centralized, hierarchical control of religious consciousness and, by extension, to undermine political and social control. We have some indication that where peasant shamans were permitted to use drug plants and were believed capable of bewitching state administrators, legitimate power would have been considered jeopardized (de Rios and Smith 1977). The use of unauthorized psychedelic substances in most societies of antiquity, therefore, would have become a crime against the commonwealth. The overview of historical use of psychedelics clearly shows a movement from open and accessible rituals for all members of society to exclusive, esoteric ones.

This appropriation of psychedelics by elite factions within societies is evident in the research published by Wasson and his colleagues in 1986 concerning the Eleusinian mysteries. This famous religious cult in the ancient Greek world influenced and inspired many of the most famous thinkers of the time. A number of scholars have suggested that the miraculous, transformative mystical visions in nine-day Eleusinian rites utilized a psychedelic potion comprised of several secret ingredients, which played a vital role in the Eleusinian Mysteries. The potion may have contained some derivatives of the poppy plant, perhaps mandrake, henbane, or opiated wines. Or Syrian rue, with chemicals similar to ayahuasca, may have been an effective potentiator (Taylor-Perry 2001).

Once higher-ranking officials in societies usurped psychedelics, knowledge of plant preparation and use quickly became extinct as cultures changed in reaction to conquest, colonialism, or more gradual pressures. The esoteric knowledge could not diffuse back to the folk level again from where it surely originated. Further, as fewer individuals took part in psychedelic ceremonies, many of the beliefs connected to such rituals disappeared or were coded in religious art, retrievable only in contemporary times through art analysis. In de Rios's work on the ancient Maya (1974), for example, she found numerous prominent depictions of the common water lily, *Nymphae ampla*. Two years later Mexican biochemist Jose Luis Diaz independently discovered that aporphine—an opiate similar to morphine—was present in the lily's rhizomes. In 1981 botanist Wílliam Emboden described the same lily's ritualistic use in ancient Egyptian civilization. Synthesis of this data supports the conclusion that *N. ampla* may have played an important psychedelic role among the ancient Maya, who—like the ancient Egyptians—placed a high value on ecstatic states as vehicles of communication with supernatural forces. We can further speculate that at the height of Mayan society's development, shamans, priests, artists, and presumably the common people all recognized and appreciated the lily's properties.

Core Characteristics in Shamanic Cultures

In 1973, de Rios prepared a report on cross-cultural use of psychedelics for the U.S. Second National Commission on Marihuana and Drug Abuse. In that monograph she described a series of recurring themes that are linked to psychedelic use in tribal societies. Let's look at some of these themes and, when possible, compare them to Janiger's volunteers' experiences.

First, de Rios noted that her participants' perception of time changed dramatically during psychedelic experiences, either slowing up to an almost imperceptible flow or racing indescribably fast. As one of the major characteristics of the sacred realm in indigenous religion is the reality of an eternal mythical present in which time is circular or reversible, the participants experienced their time distortions as evidence of spiritual consciousness. In tribal societies religious rites periodically try to reintegrate this mythical past into the present reality. Obviously, psychedelics can aid their attempts. Many of Janiger's volunteers experienced similar time distortions, as we saw in chapters 3, and some experienced them as a mystical "Eternal Now" in which time itself disappeared, as we saw in chapter 6.

De Rios's participants also consistently described spiritual animation of the psychedelic plants themselves. Many tribal groups believe that psychedelic plants possess miniscule animating spirits. We find reports in different cultures of small people of the mushroom, tiny psychedelic spirits. While Janiger's volunteers did not report this (and a natural setting was not part of the research environment), visual distortions and figure-ground relationships did shift and vary in many reports, making it appear that inanimate objects were alive.

A related visual constant was the common transformation of shamans into their animal familiars. The shaman is believed to be able to control and beckon a series of familiars for his own personal use to cure or bewitch members of his society. The sense phenomenon here is similar to morphing, in which one image remains in the mind's eye while a second one is superimposed upon it, and the first then fades away. As numerous excerpted volunteer narratives in chapter 5 illustrate, Janiger's volunteers commonly reported morphing.

Death and resurrection were also common themes in de Rios's research. Possibly connected to the dissolution of ego boundaries provoked by high doses of plant psychedelics, members of tribal societies commonly report a unity or mystical experience of oneness, conferring upon them a sense of continuity with everything that is. Called the oceanic experience by Freud, this unity may be symbolized by means of the motif of death and resurrection and may be culturally programmed by shamanic activity in traditional societies of the world. Shamans seek to induce such experiences, especially with regard to animal spirits to obtain the power and acuity that animals possess, for example, the vision of an eagle, the hunting skill of a noiseless boa constrictor moving along the forest floor, or the fertilization ability of a hummingbird. Considering the mystical experiences of Janiger's volunteers and recent evidence from neurotheologists, it seems certain that psychedelics can evoke patterns of brain activity conducive to manifesting spiritual consciousness.

A final cross-cultural theme described by de Rios was the frequency of paranormal phenomena during psychedelic ceremonies. Among indigenous people beliefs exist that psychedelic plants have the power to bestow divinatory success on individuals. However, the key element here appears to be the faith that people have in the prophetic powers of the shaman or healer, rather than any scientifically verifiable power inherent in the plants themselves. The faith of the shaman's clientele facilitates in them exceptional emotional states that the shaman uses, in what has been called the "biology of hope" (Dean 1975), to enhance clients' immune systems. In this way the healer treats clients' psychosomatic and psychogenic illnesses provoked by interpersonal and environmental stressors. Janiger's volunteers couldn't be expected to experience such paranormal activity, considering their lack of expectation or therapeutic motivation to have Janiger cure their illnesses.

Thus far the themes described by de Rios seem truly universal, transcending culture at least to the extent that their impact is readily evident in the psychedelic experiences of the most dissimilar people and in the most disparate settings. As such, these characteristics may cautiously be considered properties inherent to psychedelics and more or less reliable. However, de Rios's research also reveals three themes that illustrate how profoundly culture can influence the effects of psyche-delics: psychedelics as theater, as tools, and as sacraments. We look more closely at each of these themes in the pages that follow.

PSYCHEDELICS AS THEATER

The psychedelic experience is extremely unusual in its radically expres-sive nature, equal in force and drama to the finest theater available any-where. At the very least, there is an internal thespian flavor in the psychedelic journey, one that cannot be sensed by an outside observer. (In fact, De Rios's experience observing ayahuasca rituals both in Peru and Brazil was one of the more boring aspects of her fieldwork because all the action was internal.) However, the journey is different from the-ater since the imbiber of the psychedelic is actor, playwright, costumer, and makeup artist, even musician. Fast-moving, brilliant kaleidoscopes of colors, geometric forms, patterns, sounds, tastes, smells; fluid associa-tion of ideas; and movement are among the most unique things that most individuals have ever seen in normal waking consciousness. These are produced entirely from within the individual's psyche.

In tribal societies the culture at large and shamans share the role of stage manager, evoking one of the key characteristics de Rios discov-ered in researching psychedelic experiences among indigenous peoples: stereotypic (or patterned) visions that have specific cultural significance. That is, people reared in societies where psychedelics have been used for many centuries enter their own psychedelic dramas with certain expectations about the content and form of the experiences. Further, shamans throughout the world claim that their guidance and the music they create provoke specific, highly-valued drug visions that allow their clients to access particular supernatural entities, to view sources of witchcraft, to contact ancestors, to help the shaman heal or foretell the future, and to achieve other cultural goals. In the Amazon, for example, tribal peoples frequently had visions of the boa, believed to be the mother spirit of the ayahuasca vine. Among the Tsogana-Tsonga of Mozambique, East Africa, a common house snake that appeared to girls in Datura visions was believed to be a representation of a fertility spirit. Such stage managing also limits the danger posed by sudden, unmanaged access to the unconscious by means of a psychedelic, which is just as pivotal as its aesthetic and expressive potential. Psychodynamically-oriented researchers focus on the emotional response to such entry into the altered state in terms of somatic stress. Individuals regularly experience nausea, vomiting, diarrhea, tachycardia, and high blood pressure (de Rios 1984).

Music may be the shaman's most important tool as stage manager, and it plays a vital part in cross-cultural psychedelic use. Generally in the form of percussion but also chant and whistling, the music is considered so necessary that, for example, when the healer forgot his percussion accessories for De Rios' own experience with ayahuasca in 1968, he held up the ritual for half an hour until he was able to retrieve the rattle he used to create percussive effects during the ceremony. The shaman's music is much more important than merely setting the mood for the psychedelic experience. As noted, shamans credit it with inducing stereotypic visions to achieve predetermined goals. It also reduces the potential of negative experiences. Given the anxiety, fear, and somatic discomfort that many people experience when they have unexpected access to unconscious materials, the shaman guide creates a corpus of music that de Rios has called "the jungle gym in consciousness." The intrinsic structure of the music provides psychedelic users with a series of paths and banisters to help them negotiate their way during the psychedelic experience. Moreover, music, with its implicit structure, may provide a substitute psychic structure during potentially frightening periods of ego dissolution. Alternatively, music may facilitate the common psychedelic experience of synesthesia, or scrambling of different senses. It would appear that at the most personal level of an individual's being, namely the psychedelic experience, one's own cultural membership can determine the nature of the visionary experience.

PSYCHEDELICS AS TOOLS

Another important focus in de Rios's research, which she wrote about with Dr. Charles Grob of the Harbor/UCLA Medical Center, has been to examine the role of plant psychedelics as a tool—or in the words of Charles Tart, a psychotechnology—that allows tribal elders to control the altered states of consciousness of their adolescents by means of extreme suggestibility. In this way they can indoctrinate their youth for the purpose of survival. Specifically, psychedelic plants have historically played a major role among indigenous people in transforming adolescent boys and girls into fully participating members of adult society. In such cultures there have always been rituals to regulate psychedelic drug use and to produce what de Rios and Grob called "managed altered states of consciousness." Typically, tribal elders arrange for their adolescent boys and girls to take psychedelics, which are culturally accepted as a teaching device to prepare their youth for new adult roles.

Based on more than thirty-five years of research on psychedelic rituals worldwide, de Rios concludes that within the context of initiation rituals, psychedelics have been used to create extreme states of suggestibility to socialize adolescents by means of a fast-paced educational experience deemed necessary for their survival. Generally, and in keeping with the sociocentric character of tribal communities, the young person's psychic needs were considered less important than the needs of the social group, and in some ceremonies both boys and girls underwent great austerities and painful consciousness changes. Such rituals might include genital mutilation, sleep deprivation, and beatings in a type of aboriginal "boot camp," where young people could share and identify with cohorts upon whom physical survival in the future would often depend.

In some ceremonies psychedelics created an amnesiac state that caused individuals to have a death-and-rebirth experience, serving cultural goals of getting people to join together to be of one heart. Thus the young people would feel as if they died in their role as children and were reborn again as fully participating adult members of society, bonded with others in their age group, fully productive and eligible for marriage. More importantly, the bonding that took place during the psychedelic state ensured that participants would be generous with one other and turn to each other for help.

The extreme suggestibility properties of the psychedelic plants were central to these processes. Elders framed the behavioral patterns of their adolescents, taught them religious and secular values, and modeled appropriate emotional responses. In fact, we can say that the psychedelics were used to instill conformity in young people, which would contribute overall to group survival and harmony. In one African society, the Fang of Gabon, young men and women would be given more and more of their culture's psychedelic, Iboga, until they had the culturally desired vision (Balandier 1957). If they did not, some youths were reported to die from overdoses in their failure to measure up to their culture's expectation of their ability to experience the preternatural (Dobkin de Rios and Grob 1994, Grob and Dobkin de Rios 1992, de Rios and Smith 1977).

As coercive as these psychotechnological uses of psychedelics may appear, the Nobel Laureate, Herbert A. Simon (1990) has argued that from an evolutionary perspective it is a good thing that human beings have the ability to be docile. He calls this "bounded rationality." By being receptive to social influence human beings are able to adapt to their environment. In the challenging landscapes of tribal societies, psychedelics thus can be seen to function as powerful tools for survival, creating docile states in their youth that are at once necessary and life affirming.

PSYCHEDELICS AS SACRAMENTS

De Rios's early work in South America demonstrated the social importance of psychedelics as a form of theater for healing and as tools for initiation. In this section, we examine three contemporary subcultures to reveal a third important theme: psychedelics as sacraments. To paraphrase *Webster's*, a *sacrament* is a ritual that opens the door for people to receive divine assistance (grace) for regeneration or healing.

Among members of the Native American Church, among the Huichol Indians of Western Mexico, and among adherents of a Brazilian church called the União do Vegetal (UDV), psychedelics play a sacramental role. It is no coincidence that in many cases these three subcultures can be said to consist of beleaguered individuals. In each case the ceremonies described are part of a larger attempt to help the members of marginalized subcultures to maintain or regain cultural identity and personal well-being or to heal from the consequences of acculturation or fast-paced culture change.

The Native American Church and Peyotism

The modern use of peyote *(Lophophora williamsii)*, a hallucinogenic cactus, originated in Central Mexico and spread to southern Texas by the
1870s. More than a century ago the use of peyote eventually led to the
foundation of the Native American Church (NAC), which is the largest
pan-Native American religion in North America and has been using
peyote in rituals since its inception. It is estimated that a quarter of a
million Native Americans have been involved with this church, with
the strongest representation in the Southwest and Midwestern United
States. Garbarino and Sasso (1994) point out that the Peyote Religion
combines elements of the vision quest, a belief in the general supernatural power, and the Christian trinity. Its doctrine teaches that God is a
great spirit and Jesus is a guardian spirit. Morality and ethics are also
derived from the Judeo-Christian tradition. Some scholars would argue
that the church is a response to cultural/community dislocation and its
attendant problems. Generally, the church focuses on holistic health and
harmony with nature. In response to the severity of alcoholism among
Native Americans, the church also prohibits alcohol use and promotes
the sacrament of peyote ingestion as a powerful treatment for alcoholism (although LaBarre [1989] argues that the antagonism between
peyote and alcohol is not proven).

Within the NAC peyotism is a spiritual approach to facilitating a
sense of identity, groundedness, connection, and belonging. The peyote
plant itself is a spineless cactus with a rounded top surface that appears
above the soil. It is cut off and dried and becomes a peyote button,
which is ingested during peyote rituals. Church members believe that
their medicine functions sacramentally by allowing them to see the
truth about their lives and connects them to the peyote spirit, who will
give them guidance and direction. Organized for people who are in
need of healing from alcohol and drug addiction and who are personally motivated to change, peyote meetings are powerful rituals that pro-
mote individual introspection, group interaction, and healing in three
ways: 1) they are led by a powerful leader or guide, 2) benefit is derived
from the actual ritual or group marathon session in the form of
strengthening social networks, and 3) healing benefits are derived from
the psychotropic substance that is used as a nonspecific facilitator. The

following quote is applicable to all peyote use among Native Americans: "The peyote ceremonies are not given for the pleasure of eating the plant, but to cure some disease" (LaBarre 1989).

During peyote rituals, it is common to hear testimonial accounts of various psychological, physical, and emotional maladies being lifted by the healing powers of the ceremony. Members report altered states of consciousness that provide a fast-paced educational and redemptive experience, and youth learn community values, beliefs, and their religious traditions. Often paraphrased is a peyotist comment about how the White Man goes into his church and *prays* to God, while the Indian goes into his church and talks directly *to* God. The shamanic value of direct and personal communication with deity is enhanced by the entheogenic properties of the peyote plant. The complex hierarchy of church positions in the NAC allows Native Americans to have a parallel status structure for sincere and hard-working church members of the community. Many members report retrievals of their self-worth.

While studies have shown the positive effects of peyote on mental, physical, and social well-being (Bergman 1971), the NAC's beneficial experience with using peyote may be due as much to the context of the use as to the substance itself. As do other psychedelics, peyote makes individuals more susceptible to suggestion and cathartic expression and breaks down systems of denial. Further, peyote and like substances are "psychointegrator plants," which integrate mind, body, spirit, and emotion (Winkelman 2000). These attributes can be used to good advantage in the safe, socially sanctioned religious settings that function to focus the outcomes of the experience and to support individuals during the ceremonies. Moreover, participants in peyote meetings often form new "families" whose lives are intertwined and who provide ongoing support systems. Both early reports and recent studies emphasize the importance suggestibility plays in the context of the meetings in accounting for their positive effects (Calabrese 1997; Halpern 1996; Pascarosa and Futterman 1976; Albaugh and Anderson 1974).

Ironically, given the ban on peyote use since 1997 when the Supreme Court overturned the Religious Freedom Restitution Act, psychiatrist Karl Menninger's early comments went unnoticed when he wrote that peyote was not harmful to Native Americans, but was "beneficial, comforting, inspiring and spiritually nourishing" (1971). Based on his review of numerous studies, Menninger concluded that "[peyote] was a better antidote to alcohol than anything the missionaries, the White man, the American Medical Association and the Public Health Services have come up with" (ibid).

The Huichol Indians of Western Mexico

The Huichol Indians of Western Mexico also have a long history of peyote use. These agricultural peoples live in the Sierra Madre Occidental Mountains of Mexico. Peyote is the focus of Huichol religious and emotional life in an annual cycle of communal and extended family ceremonial and religious activity. Stacy Schaefer (1996) wrote that peyote for the Huichol "serves as an enculturating force, which echoes religious tenets and re-occurring themes that are transcended to visions, the spoken word, through myths and songs, actions and rituals and ceremonies and beliefs that permeate all levels of individual and collective consciousness." Thus participating in sacred peyote rituals is essential to being Huichol. In these rituals, the ordinary boundaries between the past and present vanish and the gods, ancestors, and events of Huichol mythic history become a physical and emotional reality. The Huichol undertake a pilgrimage to sacred lands in the Sierra Madre Occidental Mountains to acquire the plant.

Recent Mexican government action has intended to legitimize peyote use in Huichol religion and ritual. The decree would guarantee the Huichol unrestricted access to more than 182,000 acres in San Luis Potosi for gathering the plant and for holding peyote ceremonies in sacred places. However, the policy of the Mexican government has been generally unenlightened, intended to coerce acculturation and to dismantle the cultural ethos and ideological and juridical structure of the Huichol Indians. The use of the peyote appears to be pivotal in the continuing profound pride that the Huichol maintain in their culture despite these governmental attempts at cultural annihilation. Although the Huichol people have allies among the National Indigenist Institute and internationally, given the reach of the North American war on drugs, it is unclear how well they will be able to maintain their religious ceremonies, which gravitate around the gathering of peyote, the hunting of the sacred deer, and the planting of maize. Let us hope that they will be able to continue the spiritual practices that give meaning to their existence.

The União do Vegetal and Ayahuasca

Since prehistoric times ayahuasca has been used in South America to ascertain the causes of illness, to locate lost or stolen objects, to communicate with the spirits of animals and plants for healing, to allow the shaman to travel into realms normally invisible, and to initiate people into their tribal cultures. Thus it has always served socially-integrative and world-sustaining functions.

The ayahuasca drink is made by boiling the stems of the *Banisteriopsis caapi* vine together with leaves of *Psychotria viridis*. Other plants are often mixed in as well. In Brazil the União do Vegetal (UDV) utilizes the psychedelic ayahuasca as a sacrament.

Widely used in the Amazon, ayahuasca was taken up by Mestizos during the Colonial period in the eighteenth century, when the colonists lived in proximity to tribal peoples and adapted it for their own needs, frequently mixing native contexts of use with non-native elements (de Rios 1984). As a result a number of different religious movements incorporated ayahuasca into their doctrines and disciplines. Today there are several different ayahuasca churches that combine traditional, African, and Christian elements in their patterns of use.

One of the new churches, the UDV, was founded in 1961 by Jose Gabriel Costa in Brazil, where the traditional rural agrarian economy has been largely replaced since the 1950s by a technologically-oriented, urban industrial system. This shift caused massive dislocations as large numbers of unemployed rural persons migrated to urban centers in search of jobs. Urban life severely weakened the large extended family systems (Freyre 1959). In the midst of such radical sociocultural transformation, sociopsychological stress became widespread as people attempted to cope, and drug abuse became rampant in large Brazilian cities like Manaus, Sao Paulo, and Rio de Janeiro. In response new religions such as the UDV and older ones, such as Umbanda and Candomblé, proliferated to help people solve their personal difficulties. Like the Native American Church, the UDV may thus be seen as an attempt to restore personal, family, and social stability in a rapidly changing world.

Today the UDV numbers more than seven thousand members in sixty *nucleos,* or churches, all over Brazil and in the United States and Europe. Members care for the church's sick and elderly, provide food and shelter for women and children, and are actively involved in many ecological projects. Drawing on the beneficial potential of ayahuasca, members typically ingest about 100 ml. of a tea made from *Banisteriopsis caapi* and *Psychotria viridis* (with no other admixtures) twice a month in ceremonial settings, and the church was primarily responsible for the 1987 legalization of ayahuasca when used in religious context in Brazil. The ayahuasca rituals of the UDV differ from those described earlier in the chapter in terms of the sheer numbers of participants in the church ceremonies, which average around seventy to eighty persons a night. Church elders, called *mestres,* are present and commercially-recorded Brazilian music is played.

UDV adherents call ayahuasca by its Portuguese name, *hoasca.* In a pilot study in the early 1990s conducted by an international multidisciplinary team of investigators (see Grob et al 1996; McKenna et al. 1998), a group of fifteen ayahuasca-using members were compared to a matched non drug-using group of Brazilians who had no contact with the UDV. Many of the individuals in the ayahuasca-using group reported a variety of pervasive dysfunctional behaviors prior to their entry into the church. Eleven individuals reported having a history of moderate to severe alcohol use, and five of them reported episodes of bingeing associated with violent behavior. Two had been jailed because of their violence. Four individuals also reported having abused other drugs, including cocaine and amphetamines. Eight of the eleven men with prior histories of alcohol and other drug use and misuse had also been addicted to nicotine. Additional self-descriptors prior to entry included impulsive, disrespectful, angry, aggressive, oppositional, rebellious, irresponsible, alienated, and unsuccessful.

Life-story interviews revealed that eleven of the fifteen individuals believed that the ritual use of hoasca had had a profound impact on the course of their lives. Many reported an experience in common: While in induced altered states of consciousness, they saw themselves on a self-destructive path that would lead to their demise unless they radically changed their personal conduct and orientation. Many also reported encountering the founder of the UDV, Gabriel da Costa, while in the throes of a nightmarish visionary experience and being delivered by him from their terrors. Consistently, the members reported that their lives had changed dramatically since entering the UDV. Not only did they report discontinuing alcohol, cigarettes, and other drugs, but they also emphatically stated that their daily conduct and orientation to the world around them had undergone radical restructuring. They practiced good deeds, watched their words, and had developed a respect for nature. Overall, the participants reported that they had gained a profound sense of meaning and coherence in their lives.

Moreover, all eleven of the group of fifteen ayahuasca-using individuals who had prior involvement with alcohol achieved complete abstinence shortly after their affiliation with the UDV. In her visit to Manaus, Brazil, in 1997, de Rios interviewed twelve mestres and found this pattern to hold among the congregations of most of the religious functionaries in the UDV church according to their self-reports.

OF STAGE MANAGERS AND SCIENTISTS

De Rios's research suggests that where psychedelic experiences are ritualized and managed they consistently exhibit psychotechnological and sacramental potential. Janiger's experiments, by contrast, are notable for their lack of ritualism and external direction. While shamans go to great lengths to stage manage productions, Janiger refused the role of managing volunteers' LSD states and preferred to use a natural history approach in designing his LSD study. Pertinently, he was very careful to be noncommittal about music, supplying a range of recordings and allowing individuals to bring along any records that they might wish to listen to. Many volunteers chose not listen to music at all. It is interesting that all the volunteers who did listen to music agreed that it influenced their experience, affecting all of their senses, including taste and tactility. Some volunteers wrote about the wondrous taste of coffee or tea. Others saw unknown faces in the grain of wood on a door or the bark of a tree. Many had hypersensitive skin. Some people described distinctive odors. Many heard voices. But stereotypic visions did not emerge. In its place, we find the American pattern to be idiosyncratic, a peculiarity of the individual, his prior life experiences, values, beliefs, and temperament.

Janiger, of course, trusted that his research model would reveal an inherent pattern of experience based solely on LSD's chemical properties rather than on cultural expectations. As we have seen, patterns can be very distinctive, such as the mother spirit of ayahuasca reported again and again by Amazonian men and women. That the results of Janiger's study should be characterized by idiosyncracy, or distinctiveness peculiar to each individual himself or herself, is in keeping with patterns in Western society, where individual primacy is critical. Many of Janiger's volunteers, probably because they were deprived of guidance and the stabilizing support of music, emphasized somatic symptoms and unique visions; only rarely did they feel initiated into a collective group membership or healed by a sacramental experience. Creatures of Western "rugged individualism," for most the goals were self-knowledge and self-discovery, while some hoped for help in their psychotherapeutic journeys. Their LSD experiences produced what their culture proscribed, which for them was an extraordinary and unique moment.

Yet despite the major differences between Janiger's and de Rios' data sets, telling similarities do emerge. Animism of nature and objects is found in both samples, and vibratory energy is reported in all groups. At high dosage levels, the hidden or critical observer was obliterated and pure sensory data reigned. There was some degree of group cohesion and bonding, whether among the UDV members in Brazil or among the volunteers who participated in Janiger's group experiment. When people were prepared for or had an individual proclivity toward spiritual life, the LSD-like experience could provide entry into another dimension, a special place or sanctuary with significant meanings. In all cases, these powerful chemicals created a highly suggestible state in those who imbibed—a state so powerful that even in Janiger's data set where there was little if any expectation of effects, some volunteers reported an almost hypnotic compulsion to execute suggestions, even when none were given!

De Rios's personal experience with the Peruvian plant psychedelic ayahuasca neatly exemplifies both the universal and culturally-influenced characteristics of psychedelic effects. In her book *Visionary Vine* (1984) she described a stereotypic vision that she experienced—with a little variation from type. In cultures where snakes are said to be the mother spirit of the ayahuasca vine, most participants in ayahuasca rituals report seeing snakes. As de Rios was raised in an urban environment, she had never really seen snakes up close. Even under a shaman's guidance during her ceremony, no snake came down the path she was taking. Instead, she saw trick-and-treat demons from her childhood, rather whimsical and fun.

The LSD experiment conducted by Janiger, despite its weaknesses in light of contemporary research protocols, has an important place in the history of consciousness, in showing what anthropologists have argued for many years—namely the universality of the human condition, the psychic unity of humankind. What better way to test this than by holding constant plant and chemical materials, observing their effects on a wide variety of peoples, and examining the similarities and differences that emerge. Thank you, Dr. Janiger, for this legacy.

The experiments also have a legitimate place in the anthropology of psychedelic experience, demonstrating less that LSD is an uncontrollable, thus potentially dangerous, chemical than that it is responsive to the culture in which it is used. As an anthropologist de Rios has always been fascinated by the way that Westerners refuse to acknowledge the important role of psychedelics in human history, ignoring the evidence that they have been used successfully to enhance perception and intuition and have played important roles in healing and providing access to supernatural power and spiritual consciousness. These plants appear to have an enormous potential to create hypersuggestible states that can be used to mold at-risk youth to patterns of pro-social behavior, while contributing to the survivability of the community.

Let's turn now to a discussion of what the future holds for psychedelic research.

8

THE FUTURE OF LSD: THE REDEMPTIVE PATH

SINCE THE 1960s most formal clinical research on psychedelics has been at a standstill in the United States, with a few exceptions. The Maryland Psychiatric Research Center, for example, retained its mandate to study psychedelics as adjuncts to psychotherapy until 1976 (Yensen and Dryer 1997). Otherwise, however, new data in the field has been limited almost exclusively to anecdotal reports and anthropological reports like de Rios's of current psychedelic use among Amazonian patients in semirural environments (Dobkin de Rios 1972, 1984). There has, however, been rampant use of hallucinogens among the unprepared, including the youth culture during the 1960s, who saw LSD use as a tool for social change, and the more recently disaffected, who prefer such drug substitutions as ecstasy, which is lethal and dangerous, and LSD mixed with Paramethoxy methamphetamine. The last thirty years have also seen the growth in developing countries of a phenomenon that de Rios has called "drug tourism" in response to the demands of Western men and women whose search for spirituality has led them to look for drug experiences abroad (see de Rios 1994). Generally knowledgeable, these people are taken in small groups by Western tour guides to distant, exotic places where they participate in drug rituals among so-called native shamans or witch doctors. This is what one Peruvian psychiatrist long ago called "charlatan psychiatry" (Seguin 1970), a tradition in Latin America of nonauthentic folk healers with malicious and fraudulent intention who provide psychedelic plant drugs in ritual settings for their own gain. Such unscrupulous practitioners use the plants nontraditionally, exploit their victims, and are conscious of the farce in which they are involved. There are numerous psychological casualties, which de Rios and Rumrrill are currently documenting in a book to be published in 2004. As we know, the social context of drug use is a critical determinant for its outcome. Both ill-prepared individuals with little information, taking LSD or other hallucinogens mixed with alcohol or other substances, and the well-prepared given psychedelics in unpleasant circumstances will likely suffer severe adverse reactions.

It is very clear that LSD has an abuse potential; to wit, the "turn on, tune out" approach of the 1960s and the runaway use by young people during that period. It is also clear that LSD poses significant risks to users, as attested by the reports throughout this book and the frequency of "bad trips" that characterized the height of the LSD phenomenon in the United States thirty years ago. Unfortunately, the U.S. response to these real dangers has been to conduct its problematic War on Drugs, the main effects of which have been to criminalize individuals who are involved in victimless crimes, to develop black-market drug use, and to deprive society of understanding the effects of potentially beneficial substances. Ironically, the War on Drugs has facilitated the use of LSD by young, uneducated individuals prone to excessive risk, who conduct their self-experiments under adverse circumstances and without guidance. This phenomenon is, of course, the polar opposite of the practices utilized by even the earliest LSD researchers and legitimate shamans who clearly fathomed the importance of structuring the psychedelic experience to maximize its benefits and minimize its negative effects. We have clearly witnessed the failure of regulating the LSD-like drugs over the last three decades, as evidenced by the annual NIDA drug surveys in high schools, which make it clear just how available these substances are to the average teen.

The history of LSD becomes especially poignant when we consider the early promise it showed in clinical research and the fact that, compared to psychiatric drugs in current use, LSD has a safety profile of acceptable magnitude as an adjunct to mental health treatment. Despite the fear that LSD and other hallucinogens are a menace to public safety and cultural stability, when used appropriately in a clinical setting their risks are considerably less problematic than, for example, lithium, a substance used for the psychiatric disorder of mania. That medication in excessive dosages can lead to toxicity, confusion, lethargy, thyroid abnormalities, and kidney problems. Psychiatrists who prescribe the widely used antipsychotic drugs, or neuroleptics, have to be careful about inducing tardive dyskinesia, a disease that causes rigid body movements and tics in patients. Even the seemingly innocuous (and enthusiastically prescribed) antidepressive medications regularly cause daytime sedation and diminished libido.

The question that faces us now is whether we are ready to examine LSD anew, without a political agenda, in order to fully understand both its risks and its benefits. Thanks to pioneering researchers such as Oscar Janiger and more recent anthropological studies, we now understand much more about the properties of LSD-like substances and the set and setting in which they have been used effectively than was known when clinical research virtually ceased in 1962. Further, the old players such as Leary have exited the stage and taken their antagonisms with them. In place of the reckless behavior of people like Leary, a new generation of researchers has come of age and, certainly in Europe, an enlightened public policy about the potential of LSD-like drugs has emerged. Recent FDA approval of Charles Grob's proposal to research psilocybin's effectiveness as an aid for end-stage cancer patients suffering from overwhelming existential anxiety is a sign of social change even in this country. The time seems ripe to reexamine the evidence of psychedelics' therapeutic, spiritual, and creative potential in order to propose a wiser future for substances so full of promise.

PSYCHOTHERAPEUTIC PROMISE

Psychologists typically attribute LSD's general psychotherapeutic potential to several core characteristics of the LSD experience: 1) the disintegration of ego boundaries that increases rapport between therapist and client, enhances suggestibility, and releases clients from confining world views; 2) the "reliving" of forgotten or repressed memories; 3) the clarity with which clients remember their insights while under the influence of LSD; and 4) a certain dissociation from self that allows clients to analyze emerging material more effectively because they are detached from it, thus not so prone to be overwhelmed or restricted by guilt (see Hofmann 1980 and Brescher 1972). Under the guidance of able therapists, these properties are thought to channel treatment and shorten its duration—*not* because LSD is a "medication" that obscures symptoms and hides psychological conflicts (as tranquilizers do), but rather precisely because it reveals problems so clearly, increasing the potential for their treatment.

As LSD studies proliferated in the 1950s, two therapeutic models emerged. European researchers tended to use a "psycholytic" model designed to decrease psychic tension and resolve psychological conflicts by administering moderate doses over the course of several regularly scheduled sessions. These sessions were followed with group discussions and expression therapy (such as drawing and painting). North American researchers tended to use "psychedelic therapy" designed to "induce a mystical/religious experience as a starting point for restructuring the [participant's] personality" (Hofmann 1980) by administering a single high dose of LSD to intensively prepared participants. Even when we take into consideration the fact that almost all early research was hampered by poor methodologies, it is clear that both approaches yielded startling results. They indicate that LSD-like drugs are therapeutically poised to help in refractory illnesses such as drug addiction, alcoholism, and chronic post-traumatic stress disorders and in the overwhelming existential anxiety associated with end-stage medical illness, as well as with depression, alienation, and some personality disorders.

Alcoholism and Addiction

In the 1950s and 1960s several research centers in the United States, Canada, and Czechoslovakia investigated the use of LSD to treat alcoholism, a condition that has responded very poorly to other medical and psychosocial interventions. As early as 1952 Canadian researchers Abram Hoffer and Humphrey Osmond—following the then-popular

psychotomimetic model that claimed LSD could induce "model psychoses"—experimented with LSD's capacity to simulate the psychological effects of *delerium tremens,* precipitating abstinence through a
powerful and severely unpleasant psychic experience. While Hoffer and
Osmond inevitably discovered what other researchers who adhered to
the psychomimentic model were finding (namely, that LSD does not
induce model psychoses), enough participants nonetheless changed
their drinking patterns or abstained altogether to impel further investigation. Extensive and limited studies ensued at such research centers as
the Spring Grove Hospital in Maryland, the Hollywood Hospital in
British Columbia, and the Psychiatric Research Institute in Prague,
where evidence mounted that both a single high dose of LSD (the psychedelic therapy model) or serial LSD sessions (the psycholytic model)
were extremely effective in interrupting addictive patterns or instigat-
ing abstinence. When all the numbers from old reports have been
crunched (and poor methodologies considered), psychedelic therapy
claims no less than a 33 percent success rate in either significantly
reducing drinking patterns or inducing lasting sobriety (Hoffer 1970).
However, this should not be construed to suggest that LSD therapy is
some sort of magic bullet. While transcendental experiences may provide a psychological framework that facilitates recovery, addicts must
still do the hard work of coping with physiological cravings and personal feelings of inadequacy.

Under the direction of Sanford Unger the Spring Grove team
attributed their positive data most directly to their participants' experience of cosmic consciousness (what chapter 6 called the absolute unity
of being) while under the influence of large doses (200 mcg.) of LSD,
which made them more able to understand that they craved transcendence rather than intoxication and that alcohol could offer them no more
than a superficial likeness of unity. Interestingly, in the Spring Grove studies—which included cancer patients, mental health workers, and people
suffering neuroses—alcoholics and heroin addicts reported the greatest
number of mystical experiences (Grof and Halifax 1977). By facilitating a transendent mystical state in the individual, LSD thus appeared to
be an unexpected tool for helping people who suffer addiction.

Pain Treatment and End-Stage Medical Illnesses

Approximately ten years after Hoffer and Osmond began their work with alcoholics, Chicago anesthesiologist Eric Kast began experimenting with LSD in hopes of finding an effective analgesic for intractable pain because of LSD's reputation for distorting body image, decreasing boundaries of the self, and interfering with concentration, particularly the mind's capacity to selectively attend to physiological sensations (Grof and Halifax 1977). Working with more than 250 end-stage cancer patients in successive studies, Kast concluded by 1966 not only that moderate single doses of LSD (100 mcg.) were more effective than the established medications Dilaudid and Demerol in reducing participants' pain, but also that the LSD experience radically improved their mental states. Specifically, participants reported a "happy, oceanic" feeling that often lasted up to twelve days and that Kast credited with reawakening their "zest for life," reducing anxiety, depression, and fear of death, enhancing their morale, and improving their responsiveness to others.

Over the next decade Kast's conclusions were largely confirmed by research centers in Czechoslovakia, California, and Maryland, where such researchers as Stanislav Grof, Sidney Cohen, and Walter Pahnke corroborated Kast's initial findings, once more locating LSD's dramatic potential for helping people—in these cases to face death fearlessly and peacefully—in the transcendent and unitive experiences it induced.

Anxiety, Depression, Autism, and the Nature of Psychoses

Among the many hundred early research reports lie other tantalizing claims of LSD's healing potential. After years of conducting a variety of studies, the Spring Grove researchers concluded that the two symptoms that responded best to psychedelic therapy were anxiety and depression (Grof and Halifax 1977). Robert Mogar and Robert Aldrich's review of seven admittedly flawed studies of LSD's effect on autistic children between 1960 and 1966 nevertheless concluded that psychedelic therapy effectively improved the children's speech, behavior, and morale, increased their emotional responsiveness, and decreased their compulsive and ritualistic behavior (1967). And even after psychologists realized that LSD does not induce model psychoses, they advocated its use as a training tool for mental-health professionals. Given LSD's capacity to facilitate radically altered states of consciousness that could give insight into the nature of psychoses, the argument went, mental-health professionals who completed either psycholytic or psychedelic therapy could better understand and empathize with their clients, especially those with severe psychotic disorders (Hofmann 1980).

THE WISDOM OF ALTERED STATES: CREATIVITY, SPIRITUALITY, AND CONSCIOUSNESS

It is vital to remember that we are not arguing that LSD can fulfill its therapeutic promise by itself. Rather, we cannot emphasize frequently enough the necessity of a therapeutic context for directing the psychedelic experience toward meaningful and beneficial ends. As both clinical and anthropological research have shown, knowledgeable, proactive guides must be present to provide structure and/or ritual to minimize adverse reactions during the experience and contextualize experiences within larger frameworks afterward. In clinical contexts it is the guide's role to develop a therapeutic plan that both prepares clients for radically altering their consciousness and helps them afterward to work through materials encountered in the sessions. In ritualistic contexts it is likewise the shaman's or guide's role to prepare participants for their experiences, provide structure—often music—during the ritual, and help participants find healing or relevance afterward. Thus while we laud Janiger's research model of minimal intervention for the understanding it gives us of the breadth of LSD effects, we recognize its insufficiency as a therapeutic model—and, naturally, so did Janiger, who expressly and repeatedly denied that the goal of his research was therapeutic. Nevertheless, his volunteers clearly recognized the psychological benefits of their experiences and identified therapeutic potential as a core characteristic.

It is likely that the mental-health field in Western cultures is more conducive now to using psychedelic therapy successfully than it has ever been. (See Grof 1994.) Psychotherapy in the 1950s and '60s was limited by the privilege it extended to rational consciousness. Not only were nonrational states equated with pathology, but also treatment sessions were disciplined, rational affairs in which intense emotions or unusual behavior were considered to violate therapeutic protocol. In contrast, many psychotherapeutic approaches today encourage clients to tap other states of consciousness during sessions (through regression, bodywork, or hypnosis) to provide material believed to be essential for treatment. In this psychotherapeutic context LSD's potential to alter consciousness, specifically to provide access to creative and spiritual consciousness (as seen in chapters 5 and 6), can be seen as a tool for discovering wisdom.

As Janiger's work with his sample of artists has shown, the enormous flow of ideas, juxtapositions, memory recall, fierce colors, and novel forms available during LSD experiences deconditions people, allowing them to break free of perceptual ruts and creatively synthesize new ways of seeing themselves and their world. As stated earlier, Janiger did not believe that LSD enhanced creativity; rather he believed—and his volunteers' reports seem to bear out—that it allows people to access normally inaccessible parts of themselves, other states of consciousness that perceive reality differently, convincingly, and affirmingly. The artwork in the insert following page 118 speaks for this experience. When encountered by prepared minds in therapeutic settings, such creative states of consciousness also hold the promise of aiding clients caught in harmful behavior or neuroses by allowing them to experience as real— and thereby to enact—new ways of being.

LSD's therapeutic promise seems also to hinge on its relationship to spiritual consciousness. As we have seen, the role of the LSD-like chemicals in highlighting and heightening mystical operators in the brain to create the subjective experiences that we as human beings have coded as spiritual is a matter of speculation. However, comparison of LSD peak experiences and mystical states—combined with the flurry of reports from neurotheologists who are mapping neural structures that give rise to religious experiences—indicate that psychedelics may well induce unitive states of consciousness capable of changing people's lives. Certainly, organized religious groups that do not incorporate these substances as sacraments will oppose this conclusion and see evil forces at work. Yet we know from historical studies that LSD-like substances have a very long history of use in human society and are almost everywhere incorporated into religious beliefs and rituals. We also know from the case studies of the Native American Church and União do Vegetal that psychedelics used sacramentally in supportive contexts seem to show good results in reducing addictive behavior and reintegrating people into functional communities. The end-stage medical illness studies cited above suggest how powerful LSD, in particular, can be in evoking a spiritual experience that produces radical, beneficial change in people's lives.

If we admit that wisdom has its source not only in rational consciousness, we can perhaps see that the so-called diabolic drugs of abuse—the LSD substances—could play a role in effective psychotherapeutic treatments and the personal growth of individuals. As an analysis of the data collected by Janiger demonstrates, expansion of creative and cosmic consciousness is inspiring. In the care of knowledgeable practitioners it may also be curative.

THE REDEMPTIVE PATH

Psychedelics are clearly capable of inducing shifts in perception, thought, and feeling without a concomitant lapse of memory or loss of consciousness. As we have seen, many of them have been used historically in formal religious contexts, and studies of this use suggest that the states they induce can have profoundly positive, even life-changing effects on individuals, not the least because they often provide insights into meaning and psychological dilemmas. Since these substances can produce an awesome range of experiences that encompass those of diverse religious traditions, it is only natural that their effects have often been interpreted in religious terms. Among these terms is one of the most important concepts that has been developed to explain the process by which troubled individuals can be (re)integrated into their communities: redemption, which de Rios and her colleagues Charles Grob and John Baker have researched in depth (2002). Our use of this term in our research is meant to focus on the metaphoric and not the specific religious and historical use of the term.

The concept of redemption so central to the Judeo/Christian tradition is understood by many people today as referring solely to the restoration of a person to the fellowship of God and a community of believers (see *HarperCollins Encyclopedia of Catholicism* 1995). Viewed from a broader cross-cultural perspective, however, redemption can be seen as a process that frees people from less-than-desirable states and brings or restores them to a desired state. Religious and secular interpretations of the concept may differ in terms of what they consider nondesirable and desirable states, but they essentially agree to the extent that redemption refers to a change of status that is in the best interests of the person or persons involved. Eliade (1958), speaking from the perspective of comparative religion, argues that it is redemption that makes it possible to regain paradise lost, the primordial blissful state. In Judaism the concept of redemption is closely associated with repentance; in Christianity, with the idea of asking God for forgiveness. In mystical religions, there are three main means of attaining redemption: through illumination, as in Zen Buddhism; through a dispelling of ignorance, as in Gnostic traditions and Islam; or through membership and participation in the community. In African traditional religions, the need for redemption is expressed in stories of spirits of the departed who rescue people from deadly misfortune by means of ransom. In secular terms, humans can redirect the libido and reorder the soul's powers toward a more harmonious use of the personality, which may mean either a widening or narrowing of consciousness.

Redemption in its personal aspect represents the faith in the possibility of achieving a personality that is integrated both in itself and within the community (*Encyclopedia of Judaism* 1971). It also means deliverance from those evils, external and internal, that prevent people from realizing their maximum potentialities. It occurs when people are overpowered by a personal, direct experience with their deity, who discovers them in the depth of crisis and failure. It is deliverance from frustration and, paradoxically, grants people control over themselves. A redeemed life is almost always a disciplined life. As we saw in chapter 7, the redemptive power of psychedelics is not news in other cultures. In religions like peyotism in North America and the União do Vegetal in Brazil, a "mystico-mimetic" experience—where a spiritual awakening occurs—is often felt by the members of the NAC and UDV who participate in peyote and ayahuasca sacraments, leading not only to cessation of addictive behavior but also to reintegration into the community and a better life for many individuals and their families. Some of Janiger's volunteers hinted at redemption too. Several participants who reported spiritual experiences explicitly concluded that they had reconciled old conflicts and found peace with themselves and their current place in their own lives. S.W., for example, ended his LSD experience with a vision that he "took to be God's blessing": a "mixture of a cradle and an altar" that set his mind at ease after seeing disturbing reflections of himself in the mirror. About her vision of an enchanted garden, F.D. wrote that it "proved to me that I have succeeded in working out my own philosophy of life and I am now at peace with myself. The memory of that real profound peace I found in the garden will give me added strength now—for reaching deeper into myself than I ever have before. I found a rock there, solid enough to build my whole life on."

De Rios, Grob, and Baker's recent studies have shown that redemption is a powerful force in plant hallucinogenic use. Perhaps alongside peyote and ayahuasca, the synthetic LSD, with its original root in rye ergot, has a role as medicine rather than as a destroyer of lives and hopes. Janiger's monumental studies decades ago suggest it does.

FUTURE PATHS

In different parts of the world people have long found spiritual solace and healing benefits in the LSD-like substances they encounter around them. The anthropological data shows the ways in which human beings throughout the world have harnessed these difficult plants and chemicals to serve humankind.

Those of us who study history are always amazed at the subjective experience of the pace of social change. To people waiting for social change in their cultures, time always passes too slowly. Yet the last thirty-five years are a drop in the bucket if we look at historical trends, and we are poised for change. We can imagine the future of LSD taking one of the following paths.

Enlightened governmental policy that encourages the investigation of LSD's full range of effects, both positive and negative, with the elaboration of treatment models directed at refractory mental-health conditions discussed earlier.

Socially-sanctioned models for the use of LSD-like substances based on anthropological and ethnographic data, which occurs in a pro-social environment, creating transcendent experiences in a ritual setting, perhaps similar to the Peyote Religion among the Navajo or the use of ayahuasca by members of the UDV church in Brazil.

Continuing lack of support for research and the failure to understand LSD and its possible role in society, resulting in the continuation of dangerous experimentation by uneducated and risk-taking youth, legal persecution, and unnecessary suffering of individuals who might have benefited from treatment with LSD.

Janiger envisioned a special center where enlightened individuals, prepared for an LSD journey, might partake of special experiences periodically under guidance by skilled monitors, much like the ancient Greek initiates of the Eleusinian mysteries. De Rios draws upon her recent work as a psychotherapist to try to discern some psychotherapeutic role for the LSD-like chemicals. The longer one works as a psychotherapist, the more patients one sees who suffer from intractable disorders that do not yield to pharmaceuticals or different therapeutic approaches. Any substance that has a very low potential for harm but by the same token could be used to benefit individuals may indeed have a role in the pharmacopoeia of humankind.

From the point of view of consciousness studies, it is hoped that the data from Janiger's early experiment with LSD and from cross-cultural reports of psychedelic use has shed some light on the malleability of the human mind, the subjective nature of reality, and the relationship between consciousness and health. The overall positive effects reported again and again by men and women in all walks of life are not difficult to see. The way forward, however, is fraught with emotional and political obstacles, and it is hard to say whether enough changes in law will occur in our lifetimes to enable research on psychedelics for socially beneficial purposes. Yet the evidence from other cultures and from pioneer scientists like Janiger of social and personal benefit is compelling, and it challenges us. In a world so in need of redemption, threatened by personal pain, political uncertainties, and continual low-grade warfare, we would be wise to respectfully and thoroughly investigate the promises of LSD-like substances.

Appendix I

JANIGER'S LSD FOLLOW-UP QUESTIONNAIRE

This questionnaire was sent to study participants thirty days after their LSD experience.

Follow-up Questionnaire on LSD

In answering the following questions, please feel free to discuss your reaction to LSD as objectively as possible, presenting both positive and negative evaluations. Try not to be swayed in your answers by what you feel we would or would not want you to say. The purpose of this questionnaire is to get as honest as possible an evaluation of LSD from those who have experienced it.

1. Had you had personal experience with any other hallucinogenic agent before taking LSD? If so, what?

2. Did you know anyone who had taken LSD or any similar agent? If so, what had you been told?

3. Did you have any preconceived ideas about the experience? If so, what were they? What were they based on?

4. What is your general evaluation of your experience with LSD thus far? What is the most important area of awareness you feel the drug has helped reveal to you, either from a positive or negative standpoint? (If you need more room for your answer, use the other side of the sheet.)

5. What single event or insight, if any, during the LSD experience would you consider to have been of greatest meaning to you?

6. Has any major event (e.g., divorce, change of job, etc.) occurred in your life directly as the result of LSD? If so, what?

7. In what ways, if any, do you feel LSD has changed your interpersonal relations with the following (include in your discussion such attitudes as tolerance, understanding, broad-mindedness, annoyance, and irritability)?

   a. Love object (heterosexual or homosexual).
      1. What changes, if any, have occurred in your sexual relations?

   b. Parents (or evaluation of your parents, if they are dead, or if you do not see them).

   c. Children (please indicate whether or not you are a parent).

   d. Coworkers and employers.

   e. Other people whom you have known for a long time.

   f. Other people whom you have recently met.

8. Has there been any change in the way you feel about or handle your job?

9. Have you noticed any change in any of the following feelings, and if so, what specific change or changes?

   a. Depressions: depth, frequency, duration, ability to tolerate them.

   b. Periods of happiness: intensity, frequency, duration.

   c. Anger: intensity, ability to express, ability to control, ability to get over it.

   d. Love: intensity, ability to love in general.

   e. Frustration: intensity, ability to tolerate it.

   f. Elation: intensity and duration.

   g. Anxiety: intensity, duration, ability to tolerate it.

h. Physical energy: amount and consistency.

i. Mood swings: intensity and frequency.

j. Desire or ability to be alone.

k. Ability to relax and be yourself.

l. Self-esteem: evaluation of yourself.

10. Have you noticed any difference in your interests or understanding in any of the following areas? Have you changed as a participant, creator or observer in any of the following areas:

a. Aesthetic and literary:
   1. Music
   2. Art
   3. Literature and drama

b. Natural and mathematical sciences:
   1. Physical, chemical, or mathematical sciences
   2. Biological science (including medicine)

c. Sociological sciences:
   1. Psychological (understanding human behavior)
   2. Social reform
   3. Political, e.g., national and international affairs, etc.
   4. Anthropological, e.g., other cultures, primitives, etc.

d. Philosophical
   1. Moral and ethical
   2. Other universal concepts, e.g., meaning of life, your place in relation to the rest of life, etc.
   3. Philosophies heretofore unfamiliar or unimportant to you

e. Religious:
   1. Your views or understanding of a concept of God
   2. An overview of religion, including comparison of various religions

f. Other areas of interest not mentioned above.

11. Have you noticed any increase or decrease in appetites or habits since you have taken LSD? If so, note and/or comment:

a. Sex

b. Drinking

c. Eating

d. Smoking

e. Sleeping

f. Taking drugs or other medication

g. Gambling

h. Other (specify)

12. In regard to initiative, have you noticed any change in your ability to carry through any new or old projects, and if so, what has the change been?

13. Have you noticed any consistent relationship between the type of LSD experience and dosage of the drug, amount of sleep you had the night before, your mood at the time you took LSD, or any other variable?

14. Has the person closest to you noticed any marked change in you? (Please ask this person to be as specific as possible.)

15. What changes, if any, have taken place in your sense of values (e.g., the importance to you of money, status, possessions, politics, religion, philosophy, knowledge, human relationships, etc.)?

16. What change, if any, has taken place in the kind, number, or severity of your personal problems?

    a. What physical symptoms, if any, that you had prior to your LSD experience were modified or disappeared?

    b. What physical symptoms, if any, appeared after your LSD experience, and how long did they last?

17. Have you had any one typical physiological response during the LSD experience (e.g., nausea, sore throat, chills, stomachache, etc.)

18. Since taking LSD, have you had a tendency to lapse into an LSD-like state spontaneously? If so, please comment on this.

19. Has your LSD experience increased or decreased the number or changed the kind of dreams you have been having?

20. Looking back on your LSD experience, how does it look to you now? (Put a check for each item in the column that describes it best. Check as many items as are applicable.)

	Not at all	A little	Quite a bit	Very much
A very pleasant experience				
A very unpleasant experience				
Something I would want to try again some time				
An upsetting experience				
An experience of insanity				
An experience which I regret having had				
An experience of physical discomfort and illness				
An experience which did me harm mentally				
An experience which did me harm physically				
An experience of great beauty				
The greatest thing that ever happened to me				
A noteworthy experience but difficult to describe				
A horrible experience				
An experience which helped lead me to seek psychiatric treatment				
A religious experience				
A way of feeling which I would like to have all the time				
An experience which gave me great understanding into myself and others				
An experience which I feel was of temporary benefit to me				
An experience which I feel was of lasting benefit to me				
A very disappointing experience				

	Not at all	A little	Quite a bit	Very much
An experience very much like a hangover				
An experience very much like being drunk				
An experience of being temporarily freed from all worry				
A return to the feelings of childhood				
A happy experience				
An experience like traveling to a far-off land				
An experience of a greater awareness of reality				
Other than the above (state and check)				

21.   a. LSD is an experience you would like to have (check only one):

1.__only once

2.__rarely (a few times in a lifetime)

3.__once a year or so

4.__about every 3–4 months

5.__monthly

6.__weekly

7.__other (state)

b. How do you believe LSD should be used? (Check only those that you feel apply, and double check those that apply the most.)

1.__it has no use

2.__religious purpose

3.__as an aid to psycho-therapy

4.__as a treatment

5.__exploration of one's mind

6.__contacting the ultimate reality

9.__pleasure and enjoyment

10.__gaining new meanings for life

11.__getting people to understand each other

12.__only for scientific research

13.__studying psychosis experimentally

7.__becoming aware of self   14.__extracting confession, brainwashing

8.__appreciating beauty   15.__other (state)

c. Would you take LSD again? (Check only one.)

1.__absolutely not   8.__I would, but only for science

2.__no   9.__I would not mind taking it again

3.__I would have to be paid

4.__I don't think so   10.__I would like to take it again

5.__I don't want to but would   11.__I feel it would help me
   if it were prescribed   12.__I eagerly anticipate taking
6.__possibly   it again
7.__I am neutral about taking   13.__Other (state)
   it again

d. Did you tell your friends about the experience? ___yes ___no

Did you warn them to stay away from it? ___yes ___no

Did you recommend to them that they try it? ___yes ___no

22. After taking LSD, I noted the following things that were new for me and the time that they lasted:

a.

b.

c.

d.

e.

23. If you took LSD as part of our study of its effect on creativity, please answer the following items:

a. Do you feel that artists should have this experience? Why or why not?

b. Do you think LSD could be used as an approach to the understanding and/or enhancement of creativity? If so, how? Please comment.

c. How did the LSD experience relate to the creative process in yourself?

24. If you were in psychotherapy at the time you had your LSD experi-
     ence, please answer the following questions. In doing so, try to think
     of LSD as the principal agent in changing you, rather than psy-
     chotherapy.

     a. In what ways, if any, do you feel that LSD has changed your rela-
         tionship with the following:
         1. Psychotherapist
         2. Psychotherapy group (if you are in a group)

     b. In your opinion, would LSD be as valuable without having psy-
         chotherapy in the days following the LSD experience as it would be
         with the follow-up periods of psychotherapy?

     c. Is there any value in having a trained therapist with you over having
         a sympathetic friend or companion during the LSD experience?

     d. Do you believe that your LSD experience would be just as valuable
         without having anyone in attendance, i.e., how valuable or neces-
         sary is the presence of a therapist or friend during the time that you
         are under the influence of LSD?

     e. Is psychotherapy during the actual LSD experience worth the finan-
         cial cost, or would it be equally as helpful only to discuss the session
         later in a follow-up interview?

     f. Do you believe that LSD would be of assistance to nearly everyone
         who is having psychotherapy, or do you believe its use, if any,
         should be limited? If limited, how and to whom?

     g. Do you believe that the LSD experience is of more danger or stirs
         up more conflict than it is worth?

25. Comments and summary. Please write here any information or opin-
     ions you have which were not covered by the above questions.

Name_____

Address_____

Occupation_____

Date_____

Appendix II
POETRY INSPIRED BY THE JANIGER EXPERIMENT

T.H.

> *They can't touch me there*
> *In the groins of*
> *In the loins of*
> *The me, my me*
> *Deep within*
> *Past mortal sin*
> *I want to shout*
> *What's it all about*
> *You can't be devout. So why try?*

———

> *The fulcrum moves and bends*
> *The loads*
> *Superimposed*
> *The stresses and strains*
> *Go against the grain*
> *Likewise*
> *So go I*

———

The rattles and clicks
Of the other rhythm
Supercede
The smooth slide
Of the glutineous whirl of your Strauss Walzschmaltz
No. Let it be heard.

LET US ALL BE HEARD
EACH ONE
WILL BE

—◊◊◊—

In fond self embrace
The yellow music yaws
Its way around the
Round tone (void)
In the center
Knowing blithely
Of its own destruction.

Not everyone must be touched by the
phosphorescent fires—
magenta- self enchanting

—◊◊◊—

To each a peach
From each a reach

The violent fandangle rhythms
Of the violet fandango pulse
Under all under all under all under all
The humming of the trucks
Violet exhausted and reaching
It runs runs runs runs runs RUNS

—◊◊◊—

The yellow green of my seas
Enflooding to myself
The small germ plasm
Of the me that I see
(For free) you see

The harmonies must be felt in the spinal chord of the soul

—∾—

Hold your belly
Hold your guts
Hold yourself
right inna nuts
Yourself yourself
UNSUSPECTING!

—∾—

The music is like coals of color
Each within
Glowing incandescent
Tho evanescent

Round pearls
Of sound
Globs
And dobs.
Atten-u-ayyy-shuns.
Swirls. and twirls.
Gradations.

—∾—

The little
Yellow light
In the pale green
Shell
Remains lit

While the
Purple lanterns
Explode willingly!

The sweeps of me
Through the sweet sky
Unfolding
Are kin to
The dogs barking
At their shadows
Exultant.

Increase;
Loudness;
Turn it on full:
And let us all
Turn on:
Full.

With both feet
Firmly
On the ground
I await
Awakenings
Expectantly.

Without pain
I smile
At the life
That says:
Follow!
And turn
Quietly
To that which
Holds out both arms
And breathes;

Take me!
Fuck me!
Do what you will!
For I am here
For you.

C.H.

ants
dance
romance
enhance
each other
with as little
or as much meaning
as we do

———

flowers
wither
and die
to the eye
deteriorate
return to matter
to earth
reborn
warm
other form
a new life begun
the cycle
all is one

———

here I go;
the ominous glow
outside,
and from within

soon to know,
inside
and within.

The world dances
before my eyes
bernie I want you to meet bernie
we've met once before
pleasure overwhelming

I feel I am the scent of a million lovely flowers

an ocean
the tide is trying to pull me in
I will not resist

the veils lift their haziness
and make me free

the window opens for my soul to fly out
everything alive
a warm sun embraces my all

———

coughing can be
a beautiful symphony
by me
without Tchaikovsky

I am a melody
being played on an infinite
Jews harp

go and look somewhere else
for subject matter
and what does the subject matter

for all matter is subject
to other matter
and it really doesn't matter

the artist is like a god; he creates
he gives new life
new meaning
to the meaningless
which is meaningless only because we are
trying to give it meaning in the first place

the infinite wonder of it all
and how beautiful it's constructed
wonderful thought
we can never really destroy it

we are all gods; we give
things meaning
and they give us meaning
some of which has meaning
the rest
we are not able yet to
digest.

———

man in his way
is trying to imitate
the creature
at best he is only
a poor imitator

we're playing a big game with god and let's face it
he's the parent and we're the children.

just who in the hell do we think we are

———

machines are silly things
cause they won't change
everything else is changing
they are really behind the times
the worst thing in the world to be
is a machine

———∿∿∿———

artists only are able to depict
an aspect of the infinite
wonder that is in each thing
but in their own way they
give it life
that in a way we create
like the creator
but lets face it we have a lot
to learn

———∿∿∿———

I wonder
I wonder
I wonder
why I must wonder

———∿∿∿———

look at a rock
there is so much
within that rock
and yet ask someone
what they see and they
will say a rock

a rock like everything else is endless
eternal

———∿∿∿———

we are learning our lessons in our own humble way. being taught by a teacher who is so far above us we cannot understand his ways; yet he won't let anything happen to his children, anything really bad.

the earth is our play pen
god has given us free rein of
area knowing that we will
only learn by hurting ourselves

———

I am alone in a room with my horse. I look at it and see that live things have so much more meaning.

———

we are all going to school-
crazy teacher!
the lesson is just relax, kid and I'll bring you back to all this.

the lesson in art is that we can never out variation the maker of variation

all the nonsense
begins to make sense.

How do we get back in your graces good Lord?

we didn't appreciate paradise and god is teaching us a lesson

thank God for letting me back into paradise but of course the way back is through simplicity and we have lost our simplicity

to the self nothing is ugly—all the ugliness is outside

we just don't seem to be learning our lesson

we're all on our way back to paradise

we all are pulling in the same direction and yet we're all pulling apart.

F.X.

TO MOTHER

I saw the open air, the sky.
All 180 degrees of blueness humming with life.
And when the quiet motherly peace said NO,
It's too exciting for young children
You should be nice and good and come
To mother, come with mother, come in mother
The old signs that said
A witch must not be permitted
To live
It hurt and I kept the bad men away.
In the small circle and unkempt breezes
And rare mildews of good and sufficient love
For I owe all that I am
Not
To my Mother.

QUIETLY, QUIETLY

The ashes will tremble in brown afternoons
If you scream.
The echoes in fading
Will soil that calm knit
Inherited from her mother
And all her mothers.
She will frown if you vibrate
And roar.
It is rude to want
So much of life
With passion and
The afternoons will tremble and shatter
With your thunder
Unless
You quietly and gently do what your
Mother knows best and with a
Well sharpened Butcher Knife

Remove that very rude
Reminder
That you once
Were
A man.

THE GODDESS

Without love
The violet screams
Will rend and command
The emptiness
To gape and roar
It's showers
Of flowers
Wet with decay
And edged with
Dripping flame.
The boiling
Golden light
Rushes past
Like ancient
Frozen foam
Unfolding the
Crystal night.
I listen
With despair
For the net of love
To snap me back
To now
And here
And you.

GHOSTS

The Earth is peaceful now: the centuries
Have wiped away the memories of strife.
Now all endures, eternally unchanged

And deathless—for no longer is there life.
The wind blows soft, but there are none to hear.
A million times the sun has set, unseen.
No longer song of birds, no beating wings
Where nothing ever grows, is ever green.
The tide of time, unmeasured now, sweeps on,
So long that even planets must forget.
The dreamers died millenia ago;
Their fragile works are naught but dust. And yet—

There is a haunting echo in the wind,
And from the sea, an ancient, plaintive cry—
The voices of the past, which will not still,
The ghosts of dreams too unfulfilled to die.
Still they walk the long-dead Earth, these ghosts,
These aspirations of a perished race
That once had reached in rapture for the stars,
That tamed the Sun, and sought to master space.
Still they walk, these wraiths, and still they mourn
A requiem to the past they could not save,
To those who climbed so far before they fell
And swept a planet with them to their grave.

The earth is dead; no hint of life remains
Across the changeless, blinded years—And yet
Where Man once walked the ghosts still whisper dreams
That even Death itself cannot forget.

MAN OF HUNGRY EYES

Men of hungry eyes, where look you now?
Who cares, who sighs, for you?
Will you wait forever?

Yes, and one day more!
And still another,
If this will bring me closer,

To a lover,
Who is mind.

Then we shall, shall we not, be gay?
And drink nothing all day but té.
Life is Joy, Life is Earnest,
Let us eat, drink and not tarry,
For today we die,
Die to be merry,
To be Mary,
To marry,
Too many, too much, too soon,
To care about hair or bustles or muscles,
If I love alone
And die;
For a brother,
For a father,
For a mother,
For a lover,
Who is mind.
Men of hungry eyes, where look you now?

BACK TO PARADISE

Where do I go
What do I seek
Over the meadow
Past the peak
Into the valley
Infinity
I was there
And this I did see

Gardens and angles
kiss away the night
farewell shadow
all is light

mountains and maidens
jewels dance above
everlasting song
god is love

rivers and roses
unending sun
pure reborn
all is one.

sit and muse
against the sky
on wingless wings
shapes defy
staggering everything
except the imagination

I sit here and muse
and watch the sky
nature's grandure
passes by
just a few old thoughts
my cigarette and I
and watch the ashes
gently die.

if only one could capture the glorious rapture
of this

who would spend an afternoon with me
and ponder on our sanity
smoke discuss our calamity
and how we have made pleasure
abnormality

something is driving me out of my conscious mind

ashes

clash

against the wind

light bright reflection

then join the journey off

to seek another perfection

———ɷɷ———

there is nothing so dull

banal

inane

as being 100% 20th century

American

sane

sages through the ages

seek the master plan

live in joy paradise

love your fellow man.

———ɷɷ———

Yawning need emptiness

"and memory is nothingness"

No answer lies within my eyes

And sees no shape, nor hears it name

"but all the same"

The vaporous need, like Circes' tresses

Beckons and caresses and distresses

that once again, the form made known,

Is seen as   *Meaningful.*

———ɷɷ———

Wanderer, where will you find the answer

to your need?

questioner, when will you mind the dictates

of that reed of impulse felled by intellect?

ON READING THOSE BARREN LEAVES . . .

Shucks, Hux!
Noetically, poetically
Chelifer has writ...
hermetically, genetically
Entombed within his wit.
wondering and wandering
Sundering and pondering
Weeping and reaping
those barren leaves.

ROADSIDE

I sat by the roadside,
By the side of the road
In the cool of the shade.
In the sun I watched
One who walked in the dust
Of the open road.
I looked upon him
And saw ugliness,
The narrow, shifty eye,
The mouth warped
In sour distaste
I looked upon his face,
And loved him not.

In the cool of the shade
By the side of the road
The child sat beside me.
The child sat,
Looking upon the passing one
With clear and candid eyes.

When ugliness had passed,
The child said,
"He had sad feet.

"His shoes were broken,
"and I saw blood.
"I loved him
"for his sad and weary feet."

I said nothing,
Sitting in the cool shade,
By the sun-drenched road.
But night possessed my heart.

For I had not love.
I had not understanding.
I had not seen
The feet that bled.

B.E.

LAMENT

An empty night fills its void with sadness
And speaks of a dust covered coffin full of dormant gladness.
A bell shatters one pane of gloom
And a lost moon-beam enters my pale green room.
Like a child's face masked by unfamiliar things,
The little traveler leaves, forgetting to take
Its memory of the bell that so seldom now rings.

I am as before- so often alone
I call to the night, but my lips are like stone.
Futility pervades my thought-locked brain
And makes of my mind a hazy gray rain.
Life tells me how it is and what it should be,
But the small errant unceasingly reminds
Of the hopeless incongruity.

For what does it do to a love taunted by a heaven that draws a line
Between what is here, and what should be mine?

Appendix III
SPECIAL SUBSTUDY

AS CHAPTER 2 EXPLAINED, Janiger conducted several substudies in addition to the artists' experiment during the eight years of his LSD research. This appendix describes and summarizes one such study.

THE TWINS

Janiger was fascinated by the conundrum of how identical twins would react to an LSD experience. He wondered to what degree their experiences would be similar and to what degree they would differ. The opportunity to explore this question came along when a nineteen-year-old identical twin, Maria, born of first-generation European parents (her mother was Hungarian, her father German) entered the volunteer pool. She was raised together with her sister and seven other children in a lower-middle-class home in Southern California.

In their earliest years the twins were inseparable. Both sleepwalked and wet their beds and had the same nightmare. They dressed alike until high school and shared the same bedroom, interests, and friends. In mid-childhood they established separate groups of friends, but shared the same friends again by the time they reached junior high school. At the time of their LSD experiences both girls worked as secretaries. Both bit their nails. Both were bashful.

Maria recalled herself as a nervous child who was easily exhausted. She required frequent naps and careful husbanding of her strength. She suffered from restless sleep. The most important emotional event in her early years was the chronic emotional problem that arose in relationship to her father, a poorly educated, insensitive man who was repeatedly drunk. He used vulgar language and brought strange and uncouth people into the house often amid scenes of violence and agitation. The father was not particularly interested in the twin girls and he spent little time caring for them. However, he always showed a defensive and possessive air regarding them with outsiders, calling them "my little girls." Both parents were overworked and short-tempered. The twins were often spanked with little provocation.

Maria did well academically and obtained a B average in high school. She completed two years of junior college. She was not strongly driven toward any particular goal. As a young adult she felt that a secretary's job would be satisfying until she married. She still wished for an affectionate, considerate, and sober father who really cared about her and an understanding and unhurried mother who could share her confidences.

Magda, her twin, seemed to be the family favorite. Maria always followed a bit behind, and she believed that Magda was going to be the big success in life and would probably go on to a successful career. Maria pictured herself as being less positive or stimulating and without any great ambition or striving. She didn't, however, recall any feelings of hostility or aggression toward Magda. Any hurt feelings that arose were quickly and easily mended. At the time of the LSD experience Maria was dating a well-to-do young man and anticipating marriage. She was in good physical health prior to taking LSD and did not appear unduly anxious or concerned.

Magda strongly resembled her sister but had several distinctive characteristics. She wore her hair long to the shoulders, not cut short like Maria. She was more casual and less concerned about her appearance, and she appeared more expressive and outspoken. Although the details of her early years were similar to her sister's, her focus was considerably different. There was little love lost between her father and herself. She was more inclined to be outspoken and critical of his behavior, both in her childhood and at the time of the LSD study. Although she shared with her sister the propensities for being thin and easily fatigued, she was more direct and vigorous in her manner and was undoubtedly the leader of the two. She seemed to resent Maria for clinging too tightly to her. Magda struggled to assert her independence and separate nature. She felt that her parents were very poorly mated. She related a childhood episode when her mother attempted to kill the father by putting ant poison in his sandwich. She believed that her mother had attempted suicide on one occasion.

Magda always felt that she had a definite purpose in life and often daydreamed, picturing herself as a movie star or popular singer. Her hobbies were singing and collecting mementos of stage personalities.

She felt sexually precocious since her menstruation began when she was nine years old. She showed a considerable curiosity about sexual matters, initially talking at some length with a few older girls and later supplementing her knowledge with high school hygiene classes and outside reading. After puberty Magda had many dates, but she remained a virgin. Her sexual views were frank and candidly expressed. Two important experiences stood out for her. On one occasion a relative showed her some pictures of nude women and made sexual advances toward her, which she repulsed. Also at the same age of eleven, she was in a fun house with her sister. It was very dark and spooky. Everything seemed unreal and strange. There were some boys sitting in the corner and "they looked dirty." They ran after the girls and tried to grab them. Magda looked outside a window that was barred. The sun and grass outside never looked more inviting. The girls finally managed to shake the boys off after a bad fright.

Magda's high school grades were better than her sister's, and her immediate goals shifted in junior college from teaching to being a legal secretary. Magda had no problem finding dates. She was quite popular and went steady with an older boy for several months. She felt that she always had to keep her guard up because her boyfriend seemed insistent about having sex with her and was rather demonstrative. She felt that she would not marry until she was twenty-five. At the time of the study she was interested in an older married man but realized that there would be no permanency in that relationship.

The Twins' LSD Experience and the Aftermath

The girls had very different experiences under LSD. Magda felt as if she were in a little world all her own. She experienced perceptual changes and pretty blue and red colors. Everything seemed to dance. All sorts of forms, particularly Egyptian, kept appearing like a kaleidoscope. She saw a coliseum and a movie with Egyptian costuming that filled her visual images. She became very regressive, like a young child, and urinated in bed and then on the floor, tearing at her clothing. Attempts at reassurance by the monitor brought fresh outbursts. Janiger gave her thorazine, but there was more acting out and she attempted to run into the street. Maria was brought in to calm her sister, and the young women stayed together for the rest of the afternoon. Magda kept trying to push the doors and windows open and had to be restrained forcibly on several occasions. At one point she tore the curtains down from the window, pulled the shades to pieces, and attacked the tape recorder. She broke the windowpane, cut her arm badly, and had to be taken to a local hospital for stitches.

Analyzing her LSD experience later, Magda recalled that she felt that her own house was a hospital. She believed Maria was making a fool of her. She didn't want to be around her. She wished she could keep her own things apart. In response to the questionnaire, Maria checked items indicating that the LSD experience had caused her mental harm and had been "a horrible experience." She mentioned one nightmare she had soon after the LSD experience. By contrast, Magda said that for her the experience was the greatest thing that had ever happened to her. She was pleased that her sister was not with her. She mentioned many dreams and how meaningful and insightful they were. Magda had more religious emphasis regarding questions she had about her personal life.

Maria's account was different. She felt like she was watching a movie with colored designs. She fought to keep from crying, holding things in. Maria reported that she felt suspicious when she heard Magda screaming in pain. Maria felt that she and Magda were no longer one person but independent of each other. She said, "Finally she left me and I feel relieved." Magda's recollections, on the other hand, were that she always resented Maria following her, being too close to her, wanting to *be* her. She had tried to get her sister "off her back" in junior high school.

Three months later Magda wrote to Janiger and told him that she and her sister had been living apart and they were much happier. After much deep thought and talking things out, they realized that this was for the best. For these twins the LSD experiences helped them become individuals, to follow their own paths, and to recognize their distinctiveness from each other.

Janiger summarized the study in his interview with the MAPS follow-up team, calling it one of the "outstanding sub-studies that we had." He went on to say that the twins were "very close, just alike in mannerisms; what you'd expect from very closely tied, bonded, identical twins. We put them each in different rooms, gave them the equivalent amount of LSD, and they both reacted entirely differently to the drug. One was withdrawn and quiet, and the other was very active and explosive, and talking, and even peed on the floor—a few things we didn't expect. But the point I'm certainly making is they were different. The important part is that after the experiment they both went their separate ways. Before that, they both vowed that they wouldn't get married without the other one, they wouldn't go here or there, their whole lives were intertwined. After the experiment, we got letters from them, following up, saying that one of them took a job somewhere else. In short, their lives took on individual paths."

Appendix IV

ADDITIONAL VOLUNTEER NARRATIVES

INCLUDED BELOW ARE A NUMBER of volunteers' narratives, often longer than those excerpted elsewhere in the text. They range from very positive reactions to the LSD experience to a combination of positive and negative responses, appropriate to a population of men and women who hadn't the slightest idea of what awaited them in Wilton Place, Los Angeles. The first group of reports is drawn from the general study population, and the second from practicing psychotherapy patients, who represented a small segment of the volunteers.

VOLUNTEERS IN THE GENERAL POPULATION

R.I.

I started out about one hour after ingestion, with a feeling of being joyful and powerful. I was king of the mountain. I was Las Vegas and Manhattan and big and unbeatable. But this did no good. I was completely without humor, which is something I think is extremely important to have, and I have always highly valued. Also, I was very lonely. I became a huge hawk, but my power, my beak, was trapped by a cage around myself. The cage represented loss of humor and feelings of loneliness. Then I discovered if I simply opened my beak and relaxed, I had once again a feeling of goodness, but the feeling of being powerful simply had to cease.

I then made a decision. I chose forever to give up ideas of power over myself and others in exchange for the feeling of well-being and humor. I then became an architect for the rest of the session. The rest of my session was spent in building up a concrete structure with my new resolves. I was down to the level of my subconscious. The bottom of the structure, the cornerstone was twofold. First—to thine own self be true. Second — simplicity. From there I completely sealed off all desire for power over mainly myself but also over others. For this I substituted Radar or Intuition, something I have always felt I had lacked. I also put in my structure a power to look inside, only for purposes of being able to put things into perspective by laughing at myself. This is my sense of humor. From this simple concrete edifice underground, I built top-side, a religious temple dedicated to "Thine Own Self be True." I felt like a crusader. Now I know what gives people like Billy Graham and Aimee Semple MacPherson their drive. I tried to figure out love. The only answer to what love is was given to me as "Love is Important." When I tried to delve further into love, I came up to No Trespassing signs. I then knew that if I went any further into this area, my edifice and also my bargain to myself would collapse and I would really be in bad shape when I came out of the LSD effects. So from this time until the end of the session, I kept plugging up further holes and questions with the realization that this was the only way it would work. I made only one concession to myself. There is only ONE opening in these structures as it now stands. That is an LSD opening. My inner mind is completely closed to all suggestions now and the only thing that will penetrate it will be an LSD session. This will, of course, bring down the structure, but after the rubble is cleared away from beneath the structure a new and a superior one can be built in its place.

A.C.

This volunteer participated in the birth and delivery of a small baby—herself. She went back to her first breath and each new gasp of air was a startlingly joyous experience. She felt naive to a certain degree.

I was in a good and humorous mood. I thought to myself that this felt like actual lovemaking should feel—everything inside of me was sharp with feeling and emotion. I finally decided I enjoyed it and needed it and my mind then started conceiving the idea that I was having intercourse . . . but my mind also told me there was no one there. I thought of Roger . . . my actual desires and yearnings for Roger as a mate became so strong that to a point I didn't care who it was. The first person I could find would do. I thought I would actually attack someone. It's funny, all of a sudden now I realize whether right or wrong, that sexual enjoyment can be a must, a part of living, like hunger and thirst with no feelings of love for the mate. Yet for once, lovemaking and the giving of yourself completely didn't feel like it was dirty, just a need, like breathing. Now I'm starting to see, now I know that you can love one person, husband or wife, and still have these feelings. It is not wrong, it is a blessing. This now brings to mind the other aspects of love in a marriage. Now, sex isn't the only way of showing love. It goes along with it but it isn't the predominant factor. Hurray! Now I'm free from that. This feeling going on inside of myself now takes on new meaning. I can now feel as though I can compete with any other woman. If I can just transfer these same feelings to real life. If I could accept lovemaking in real life as free as I am accepting it now, I would have no worries over the other woman. Other women be hanged and if my husband slept with her for one night he still would sleep with me, and brother, look out! I feel that no one can beat me now with this combination. I now feel no hatred towards Roger for any or all lovemaking with others. I no longer have the feeling that because he went out or kissed or had sexual relations with another girl or girls, I don't feel he did it because he didn't love me but instead because of his need. He desired and needed whatever person he was with. Maybe it's the way he was and maybe it was me. I only know that the next time it happens if and when, instead of my being hurt, I'll just feel as though the competition is getting stronger and I'd better get on the ball.

I.A.

I began to feel weak behind my knees. The wall, after an hour, began to undulate. I became aware of light filtering in through my back of my skull where formerly I felt pressure. Suddenly the light came through my entire body again, but I felt massive. My hand looked like a relief map of hills and deep cut gorges. I began to laugh because everyone's self concept including my own seemed so funny in the face of these sensations. From one viewpoint I was a dense gas, from another a highly compressed solid form, another as big and complex as a mountain . . . all depending upon the comparison being made. I went to the toilet. As I urinated, it seemed the water would never stop. Huge quantities of fluid left my body and I was shrinking and drying up. I had any somatic feelings. My left side felt chained and in a sticky gray mire. This changed over to small trickling of life that ran through me in blinking lines of light.

This housewife had a second experience a month later.

Inside myself I felt a joyful feeling of life and I glowed like a giant pillar of energy and radiance. I painted a child doing the hula-hoop. Each brush seemed to weigh several pounds. I felt the wrenching movements inside and knew exactly where to paint the first stroke. It took several seconds or minutes between strokes to get just the right color and placement. Each move was certain and final. I had no choice. There was only one right way. The picture was not beautiful. I didn't even like it. The upper left hand corner was empty and gaping. This tied in with my headaches on that side. I realized it was a picture of myself and my bodily feelings. I tried to fill in the left hand corner and broke into a sweat. I finally put down yellow there. Although my painting was finished, it looked raw.

When my husband came in and started to suggest something, I interrupted him, filled with anger. I wanted no external suggestions. The single purpose of my painting was ruined by this interruption. There was only one single line of feeling behind this painting and it had been destroyed by the uncertainty that his remark created in me. I sat while the rage went through me and then I began to paint in that rage I felt. I quit painting in a mood of frustration.

Q.A.

My own feelings amounted to an emotional catharsis. I had feelings, which I haven't had for many years. The visual imagery was incredibly beautiful. Most of the images seemed to be strangely beautiful underwater plants of a variety of beautiful shapes with colors that ranged over the spectrum of the rainbow. On a number of occasions, I laughed so inanely that I felt that my wife *deserved an explanation lest she feel I was keeping private jokes from her. There was a period of introspection. This began involuntarily. On occasions I would slip into introspection and think about myself, even though I might be trying to listen to what someone else was saying. I gained a number of insights. I experienced a feeling of inner peace and security and a sense of rapport with my unconscious, feeling self that I have experienced on all too few occasions during my life. My contacts with the others were so empathetic that I had this wonderful feeling of communicating with others that one enjoys only when he is communicating at all levels. The experience sparked me to renew my effort to let the feeling me play a bigger more important role in the relations between me and others as well as between my conscious and unconscious self.*

F.C.

I laid down. I was aware of looking at a white, textured ceiling about ten feet square with a shiny brass light fixture in the center. This brass fixture became my focal point and seemed to be a bottomless whirlpool going away from me and then the color came! The most beautiful brilliant colors I have ever seen. The first array was solid sparkling yellow covered with a fine old lace pattern of white. Next came a gorgeous green, followed by a wave of blue and then a golden rich brilliant brown. These colors cannot possibly be described in print for I have never so much as imagined colors being so beautiful or so brilliant. I was like a starving man finally being given food as I simply lay there, with my eyes wide open and wallowed in all the beauty.

. . . I remember spending some time in mortal combat with two common house flies. Their buzzing sounded as loud as jet aircraft and was definitely interfering with my hallucinations. It bothered me to such a degree that I decided to master them, by commanding them to land and be still while I let my imagination wander in the beautiful world I was in. This actually seemed to work for a while and then I felt as though I had lost control completely over these rude insects. The only explanation was that they were trained flies and had been turned loose in that room by the doctor so he could analyze my reactions to a horrible hindrance.

My recollections are that I aimlessly roamed through my newfound world of wondrous color for about three hours. Then it slowly became apparent that I could exercise some control over my visions. I decided to put this power to good use. I divided the room into four equal sections. Upper left was for my personal problems. I could see these problems as I arranged them in order of their importance, so I could take them, one at a time, and deal with them. As it turned out none of them were really problems but more like the prime interests of my life: my family, my vocation, my home, relatives and friends.

Perhaps the most profound vision was in seeing the Lord Jesus Christ, actually in all His glory, as described in the Bible. I seemed to be begging His forgiveness in forsaking Him for so long. His reaction was one of sternness but understanding. This vision was so strong, that later in the day in the company of my wife, when trying to relate to her this religious vision, I would break down and cry very heavily. I did this on two different occasions that night.

Getting back to the square, my ceiling was divided into four squares: upper left, for problems; upper right for solved problems; lower left, religion; lower right, my playground. During the whole sequence of putting my thoughts in order the problems, religion, etc., I would seem to slide off the thought into this playground. The playground was where I could just relax and enjoy the panorama of color. I would stay in this area until shocked out of it by an earthly noise, then I would go back to the problems until once again, I would eventually slide off, back into the playground. One beautiful vision, above all, stands out. Imagine a magnificent deep brilliant blue background as huge as the sky and suspended in front of it in a display that looked professionally decorated is every jewel known to man, each trying to out-sparkle the other.

I'm being completely honest when I say it's a certainty I'm a better person because of my experience with LSD. I actually solved some materialistic problems such as how to present myself and my ideas to certain persons in regard to the position I want. I even went so far as to figure out a way to drain my swimming pool without renting expensive equipment. I planned in detail the construction of a backyard patio, which had been a sticky problem. I even planned the color scheme for this patio. Another thing I saw was the finished product of remodeling my young daughter's bedroom, something I hadn't been able to decide on for weeks.

O.A.

The LSD experience was one of the most gratifying experiences I have ever had. My wife, Paula, came back into the room and asked if I would like to go *for a walk. She said it would be fun and I was agreeable. I would probably have followed any suggestion. It is not an Aristotelian universe. The ability to engage in abstract thinking is much more difficult, particularly to express one-self verbally.*

This teacher then went on to use all kinds of psychological theory to try to explain what was happening to him.

F.F.

I felt like Peter Pan in the Laughing Universe. All of it was uncontrolled laughter. I began to giggle about forty-five minutes after swallowing the dosage. I could see brightly colored spinning pinwheels. I felt as if I had been shot into outer space all of which was colored purple and green and yellow in geometric designs. The whole universe began to vibrate with laughter and then I realized that laughter had a dimension: you could see it, a jolly purple and happy green and the whole universe was laughter. Laughter simply was, it was a rhythm, a color, a frequency. Everything was laughter. I felt that laughter was infinite. There was laughter before there was anybody to laugh and there would be laughter afterward. It was not something that happened, it was a separate permanent everlasting state.

Back in his hotel room later that evening at 11:30 P.M., some ten hours after the LSD dose, the volunteer, a writer, looked for a pen, hoping he could remember enough physics to work on the formula for turning carbon and hydrogen into laughter.

He had a second LSD session a year later.

This experience was not pleasant. I felt chilly and within two hours, I was shivering. I wanted to use the state to see what I could write or draw and let the hallucination carry me where it would. Neither seemed to work very well. I was walking through a dark, giant forest. It was a Disney-like forest with menacing tree trunks and giant trees. The whole world seemed to be rather dark and cold, not particularly hostile or menacing, rather indifferent. There were other Grimm's Fairy Tale creatures: dragons, griffins, serpents, and so on. I remember thinking: are these things native to our unconscious? Does all of humanity pick the same sort of symbols? Suppose we had never read or been read these fairy tales, would we still see griffins and dragons? and the fairy tales: did they come as a result of these unconscious myths or did they produce them. It does seem to support Jung, I feel, but I'd still like to know.

The volunteer drew various animals he saw in the dark wood.

I had the feeling that one doesn't strike—when drilling into the subconscious. It's a terrific, flowing gusher of emotion every time. Some wells are dry, some bring up only salt water and this was one of those times. I felt frustrated because I felt and still feel that there was something important to discover there, something that is lingering just over the horizon, but that I had missed it. It's still there. I hope to drill again at the earliest opportunity.

H.A.

This volunteer left the building to look for a pad to write on. He stopped in a church and was conscious of the beauty of the arches which seemed to grow larger or "arch all of their archness" as he watched them.

They reminded me of whale ribs. The sun seemed to cover in great waves of light and the lantern type chandelier would enlarge as the waves hit. Above the altar was a great white plane upon which rested the crucifix. A brilliant red seemed to frame Christ. Again came the waves of enlargement and I thought how nice it was for Christ to have such a beautiful place for adornment.

After a period back in the office with laughter, his little room, which had been so adequate, now gave him a sense of foreboding and terrible claustrophobia.

The curtains swooped at me in waves, and they represented something even worse than death. I never could establish what but vaguely resembling insanity.

He became aware that the shackles binding him were society's laws and mores.

Eventually I became angry and filled with hate. I left out my anger at the need to be important, at the world's acceptance of importance.

Now feverishly I wanted to draw the beauty of the room, its objects. I began craving with great freedom and a sense of urgency about explaining the essence of these objects. I saw the beauty of an ashtray, the curtains, which I threw back to reveal a window of more beauty. The orange-pink-green-white loveliness of a pack of potato chips. I lay down and enjoyed the quiet play of the shadows of the leaves outside. I tried to decide how I could come back to the world of family and work. I never quite reached a conclusion and I really didn't want to go back. I realized that I had gone back to the beginning of time and like the children of Paradise, I didn't want to come. I felt I must explain the essence of woman and man to myself. I went to a mirror and started doing a self-portrait. I did three, the first of which was obviously the Puritanical John I hated. The third was the core of men in prisms and plants like stained glass. I drew but I was dissatisfied with most of the sketches, but finally got one that I felt was fair.

B.L.

My throat felt odd and I felt numb in my jaw. I feel like a fish swimming, flowing along. All of this life has been false; what does it all amount to, trying to make a show. You began thinking that you are all there is, then you began to think you are part of everything, with the ability to know how the creatures were made: the sea shells, the colors were rippling and flowing, all the green tentacles of shell fish blend together. All the tremors began shivering and join in opalescent light; and yourself too. You suddenly realize that you can be a part of all this. This is no point of separating yourself.

Sometimes we get false concepts of things. It is already set. You and I, orange and green, a mess of colors. . . . Pictured myself as the Buddha, looking down into a bowl at the cigarette. Why give up something pleasant? Why throw out the cigarettes? Smoking kindles the imagination. When I have had enough, throw them out. Get your mind into a heavenly state of being; not necessarily good or bad but just is, rhythms. Everything measures as light and energy; we are just in the stream of light. Light waves get on a current and soar up with it into the cathedral top.

Responding to Janiger's questionnaire some time later, the volunteer had this to say:

I am more tolerant of my wife and her individuality. There is a general rise in happiness. My elation over certain spiritual aspects since LSD have had great intensity and long duration. I am more satisfied with myself now that I have better control of myself. Better understanding, and more affection for other people as well as for myself.

God is everything. Beauty, understanding, love, affection, wisdom. I am interested in archaic patterns and images of the soul. I experienced much of this in the LSD state. My value on money has lessened. I see religion as a way of life. I am able to control my alcohol drinking now. I saw the LSD experience as very majestic. Music stimulated the action of colors and imagination. After the LSD, I lack fear; I have a better concept of love, no religious fears of God or orthodoxy, no hates or revenges, clear thinking.

I saw an existence of the spirit where human bodies do not exist, only the spirit is the creative process and it has no limits. I believe that a person could gain great mental powers through LSD.

C.D.

The first physical symptom of the drug's effect was an abrupt onset of sexual sensations in my groin, twenty minutes after taking the pills. These voluptuous feelings quickly spread. Familiar sensations of sexual excitement but strangely unaccompanied by sexual images or thoughts and unprovoked by sexual cues in the surroundings. First images that appeared after I closed my eyes and lay down were geometric designs in color, regular structures that moved slowly and reshaped like patterns in a kaleidoscope. I began to shiver with cold and needed a blanket. . . . Soon the geometric figures were replaced with scenes like theatrical sets, all of which were lit at first with garish lurid shades of green and violet. . . . When I opened my eyes, the air in the room seemed filled with a dense yellow light. Objects that I tried to focus on would dart and flutter jerkily as if the speed of a movie projector had gone out of adjustment. Nearly all objects were surrounded by an aureole of light-like objects immersed in a sunlit swimming pool. . . . People would appear with distorted heads drawn by Picasso or by Modigliani. Nearly every style of art I knew appeared at some point either in background decoration or embodied in real objects and people.

The volunteer saw scenes from different movies he knew, *An American in Paris* and *Fantasia*.

I felt slightly abashed that my visual pleasures should be simpleminded and romantic, and so heavily influenced by second-rate popular movies, but these pangs hardly diminished my childish pleasure.

He became reflective as he experienced different visual distortions.

This is how an artist feels, isolated from others, seeing visions, signs, colors and forms that others tone-deaf or color-blind to these messages simply cannot perceive. My feeling was not that I had become an artist or that I simply understood what artists have often said about their craft and their relation to the world. But that I had been privileged to see out from the skull of an artist for a limited time by this LSD. I have never been very sensitive to painting or sculpture, which have never been even comparably as important to me as writing or music. These thoughts induced a lasting change in my attitude toward artists and art. Art is all that is important in the world—a feeling not natural to me of awe and humility in the presence of the artist's rich perceptions. The artists are kings of the world. The artist is managing to hold on to, to perceive some of the raw data that is usually discarded or reshaped by the brain, some of the eye's conjectures that would normally be tested and rejected by the trained observer below the threshold of conscious perception. The normal person "knows" the colors of things, their shapes, and the way sensory perceptions should hang together, when his eye would see configurations and colors that he knows are not there. These false alarms and faulty guesses are suppressed before they ever reach consciousness. The normal observer . . . perceives consciously what is mainly true, what persists, what is sufficiently consistent with his preconceptions, but he does this by rejecting from consciousness a Babel of messages conveying wild guesses, false clues, irrelevant details including a wealth of perceptions that convey confusingly and unnecessarily for normal purposes all the ways in which this image at this moment in these surroundings differs from the similar images to which the brain has learned to equate it, including images of the same scene several moments earlier. Perhaps the artist sees more differences and different similarities of a sort not commonly useful enough to be consciously perceived, perceptions available to the normal brain but not generally admitted to consciousness. The artist rescues, for purposes of his art, messages from this Babel conveying shape, pattern, beauty. He hears music in the noise.

B.L.

I had a feeling of nausea, a feeling of undefined uneasiness which elicited clammy perspiration and a certain feeling of coldness. . . . I sat in a yoga position on the bed, after taking off my shoes. My first really impressive alteration in perception happened. Looking steadily and fixedly at a small area of the blanket . . . I observed that the most minute tufts of blanket swirled up into lovely patterns. These issuing patterns rose up from the depths configuring into highly delicate forms, which are seen markedly in ornamental Persian rugs. That's where those patterns come from, I observed.

I noticed the curved edge of the chair in the room. The chair's covering was a green, white, and yellow plaid in design. Just the rounded edge seemed to be in motion. When I went out of doors, the elevation of the ground and streets seemed distorted. I walked easily. I walked looking at the superb beauty of nature, wondering if only I and the children understood the meaning of this beatific existence. Pausing by a wall near an expansive garden, I listened to the birds singing. One voice of a bird seemed to be calling to another. Other birds answered which seemed to call forth a responding answer. Many other birds called and answered in what seemed like communication.

. . . Suddenly I became aware of a tree a short distance away. I walked toward it and then stood beside it. It had many roots pressing into the ground around its large base. The swirling configurations I had noticed in the blanket and upon the chair now seemed to appear in the roots of this tree. The tree seemed to be in process of becoming and disappearing. There were great gnarls upon its trunk. The gnarls appeared to swirl and convolute. The tree was ugly and forlorn. I spoke to it asking it not to feel badly that it was large, knuckled and hugely warted.

VOLUNTEERS FROM THE PSYCHOTHERAPY SUBGROUP

V.R.

The experience itself was utterly extraordinary. Physically, intellectually and emotionally, I was stretched fantastically beyond any ordinary experience. My body seemed to stretch completely, beyond itself as though I had two bodies and I was struggling to release myself from the other.

I was completely aware of my realistic circumstances and my immediate surroundings. I could consciously report and discuss the most intensely bizarre hallucinations with people in the room while they were taking place. I had almost total recall. My memory of the hallucinatory period, that lasted several hours, is in fact more vivid and complete than my memory of the preparatory period just before the experiment.

I gained fresh or new insight into matters of long-standing personal concern. I was able to perceive and analyze an oil painting much more sharply than I had just before I took LSD.

I think intellectual perception was stretched. My rational experience was challenged, stimulated, provoked. I was required to find reason and order in the chaotic fantasies released by the drug. When I couldn't pursue the hallucination and overtake it intellectually, I experienced intense, sometimes overwhelming, emotional reactions, abruptly closing or shifting the hallucination. Hysterical laughing or crying, inevitably linked were most common.

The hallucination, itself, was wildly brilliant, surrealistic at times, painfully naturalistic at others. At one time, I was inside a volcano about to erupt. Several times I was involved in the crucifixion of Christ as spectator, participant, or Christ himself, suffering acute pains, agonizing in fantasy, which caused no conscious physical pain whatsoever. At one point the universe quite literally shattered. I was lying down in a well-lit room with a shaded window on my left, allowing considerable diffused light to enter. I had an overhead light above me quite bright in my eyes. When I opened my eyes during the cosmic shattering fantasy, the room seemed dark and the overhead light seemed uselessly dim. When I went home I could look directly into the late afternoon sun, very blinding that day, without sunglasses or squinting my eyes. The colors I saw in the shattered universe seemed to approximate the brilliance of shattered sunlight.

The response to each of the shifting hallucinations was deeply emotional for me, as though the four-dimensional space bubble in a shattered universe of Paul Klee design were personal experiences, profoundly moving and meaningful if I could really penetrate them. I experienced human emotional reactions of joy, agony, pleasure, apprehension, exactly as if the visual fantasies were distorted images of people.

I value LSD primarily as an extraordinarily effective releasing agent. After the experience, I felt relaxed and stimulated. There were no unpleasant aftereffects. I ate well, with good appetite and slept soundly. I continue to experience a residual feeling of release, exhilaration and extended perception. I think I will continue to perceive color and shape with sharper appreciation. I am curious and responsive to all phases of nature.

As a writer, I now believe that I can write with greater confidence and ease about myself, my childhood, my parents, and my own feeling. I have an urgent and immediate desire to penetrate and understand a number of troubled areas of experience, which I have always found difficult to approach as a writer. Since the LSD experience, I can speak about such problems.

The released articulation concerns my urgent will to penetrate the unexplained, unexplored fantasy areas of personal experience. I think it has a role in psychotherapy. For me, release of poetic imagination, emotional memory and visual perception stretched fantastically beyond any previous memorized or imagined experience.

E.L.

This volunteer was nauseous and fairly sick. She vomited and was given medication to lessen the nausea.

My vision is blurry. I am lost in bulkiness. I burst into tears and cried bitterly. The nausea and the crying were so very distressing. I stopped to look at a rose bush, which was growing in front of a house. I tenderly touched a full blown pink rose and that rose seemed to me at that moment to contain all the beauty in the world. It was the essence of beauty—delicate, feminine, beautifully formed, fragrant, soft to the touch.

It was perfect. I seemed to be lost in contemplation of the rose, of its beauty. As a rose petal fell to the ground, I felt sad that I had loosened the petal from its moorings but the doctor suggested that I pick it up and take it with me. My sadness vanished as I became completely absorbed in the petal. All of a sudden I had the feeling that I wanted to use all my senses at once. I wanted to see, feel, smell all at once. The air felt good, the petal was mine and I kept caressing it with my lips as tenderly as one would a small pink helpless baby or soft lips and cheek of a sweetheart. We walked to a park. I heard voices dimly, I saw people dimly until a young slender woman in a bright red dress passed us and continued down the walk. She seemed to me femininity itself. She was graceful, slender, straight and as she walked further on, she seemed to be swaying her hips from side to side with a gentle motion as if proudly proclaiming her sex to all the world. I wished for a moment that I too could walk down a park path, in a bright red dress. Tall, slender, graceful and feeling completely feminine.

We walked on a little and the doctor pointed out a group of trees to me. I was immediately drawn to them. They were magnificent with their twisted, tortuous roots above ground. They looked as if they attained their strange shape by intense struggle, as if after crawling along the ground for a few feet, they somehow managed to push themselves into an upright position at an angle, which made them look as if for them, life was an intense struggle to straighten up. I neared the trees and was able to touch one. It seemed to contain a yielding softness, a kind of soft masculinity—strong but not brutish, soft but not too weak or too feminine. I wanted to stroke the tree and lean on it and seemed to be lost in sensory responses. I examined the bark and it was a beautiful brown and cream color. It was so soft and feathery that by rubbing it gently I was able to pull a few strands of bark away. The tree seemed to take on an aliveness, almost a human quality.

I left the park reluctantly taking a small one piece of bark with me. I now had two pieces of magical beauty in my fingers, the rose petal and the bark. The petal and the bark in my hands had a special beauty. They were precious possessions. Upstairs in the doctor's office, I reflected on my rose petal and bark. Suddenly I was overcome by a sense of sadness that such beauty was perishable, that my rose petal was now wrinkled by all my caressing and I started to sob again. The quiet and peace I felt in the park was gone. I was very distressed and I gave way to alternately crying and laughing.

The volunteer was given sodium amytal. When she returned to her home she had a feeling of well-being. She thought how wonderful it looked, so fresh, so new. The pictures looked brighter, the flowers and vases more alive, the whole house had a look of freshness. She was tired, as if she had worked hard all day.

E.N.

As a psychotherapist, I am aware of both worlds. The aspect of reality of the everyday world and the other aspect of reality commonly referred to as psychotic. LSD took me into a world so real, so perfect that my mind was constantly busy relating the two. I had an omnipotent feeling and felt compelled to take the two aspects of reality—schizoid split and somehow bring them together in a holistic concept. This was the only way myself could find true happiness.

Life's calling was for life itself, completion of the inner search—the great truth. Once one has pleasure it ceases to exist: beware of women who come to give you pleasure, for she shall indeed give you pleasure, and when she has, she will rob you of desire, leaving you empty until another aspect of the self builds a tension and the search goes on. Left alone, my feelings plummeted to absolute and complete despair. Tears and convulsions were profuse. I broke through the level of despair and ecstatic pleasure was so great as to be very painful and I screamed and yelled. Only mankind can be so greedy as to demand greater pleasure than he was meant to have. I had that intense pleasure in LSD to the degree of pain. The situation is untenable. Like starving yourself for three days to enjoy food all the more on the fourth day. I found the only reality with any validity—the cosmic experience, one with nature and God.

I fantasized the Yogi concept of absolute bliss—that would be death. Our life is based on physiological tension or dissatisfaction. Nature knows when, where how and how much. I fantasized about the end of civilization, a twinkle of light goes out in the Eternal Darkness only to spark again on another planet elsewhere as it must have been doing countless times and will do countless times in eternity.

The pattern is clear. Nature builds time clocks within creatures as well as in cultures so that civilization can go only so far, until it sows the seeds of its own destruction, or rather the ending of the tension cycle. Mankind is schizophrenic. His split is with nature. He applies the scientific principle and divides, divides until there is nothing left or builds the edifice complex tension to the bursting point and destroys himself, such as with atomic bombs or even more intelligent means.

I am God. I became as One. When God is wrong, I am wrong. When God is right, I am right. There is no right or wrong. Formal education is as buggy as the psychotic culture that produced it and with the scientific principle splits man into even smaller fragments. It is like standing in front of a barn, running around it and discovering that you had been there all the time.

Trying to resolve the two aspects of reality is like turning a light switch on and off fast enough so that it will be light and dark in a room at the same time. Then the realization comes that they are aspects of oneness, a unity, and are compatible with each other, bringing a fuller life.

The fantasy that saints are reformed shit-heels. They learn from their own wickedness. React the opposite and become saints. There is no such thing as good without its counterpart evil, so why divide that which simply is. Leave it whole as Nature-God intended.

G.L.

This volunteer was an artist inhibited in her painting. She was in psychotherapy and had had a previous LSD experience where her work underwent a change from somber to vivid. She was using pure colors with a new preference for the freshness, spontaneity, and sparkle of watercolors. On the second occasion she was left alone in the studio with her own paints and small plaster kachina doll.

Before long, I became aware of exquisite freezing cold of intensity I have never before experienced even in wintry blizzards of Michigan where I grew up. I crouched into the blanket and stayed there for hours.

The impressions raced by in such rapid succession that it is impossible to catalog or record each of them. I perceived that I was being transported with lightning speed through millions of scenes of people in the vital processes of living; living with the full gusty vigor that contains no artifice or sham or veneer. Whirling madly, I was rushed through busy city streets and squares; into festivals and celebrations, and everywhere I was acutely aware of the vivid pulsing realness of the living. I felt as if I'd seen all of life sliced clean through the middle and in the raw, gaping wound was the exposed, quivering being-ness of people.

Everything was brilliantly colored and pulsating with the warm, flowing, living quality and I was part of all of it, the crazy, chaotic mish-mash of moving whirling dancing people, buildings and landscape were yet somehow not chaos. At times, I felt torn apart by pure feeling, not an entity to be segmented into love or hate or passion or fear or any other of the myriad human emotions. It was feeling itself, at its origin before it became divided into its component parts and the force of it as so great that it burrowed deeply into the very soul of my being. Again it could not be categorized as pleasure or pain. It was pain so excruciating that it was pleasurable and pleasure so exquisite that the pain of it was agony. At another time, I felt that I went clear to the source of light, not to the sun or to any reflected source but beyond—to the actual origin, an IS LIGHT idea, which I suppose would be God but I did not think of it thus. I felt a worshipful reverent pleasure-pain.

Throughout the experience I had the disconcerting annoyance and yet enjoyment of being yanked out of what kept promising to bring the spiritual insight for which I longed by flirtatious little feminine creatures who flitted seductively across the screen of my mind, some svelte and slender in vibrating, lovely dark colors, batting eyelashes and twitching hips provocatively; others buxom in pink and blue with ostrich feathers and can-can skirts, glancing flirtatiously over soft bare shoulders. Then came Mulatto girls, Hi Yaller gals and stylized Disney-like creatures with painted eyelids and sweeping eyelashes. All were feminine, cute, provocative and flirtatious, enchantingly and appealingly naughty. While I could watch them, I was also all of them, winking, fluttering eyelashes, laughing bewitchingly and seductively and twitching hips invitingly or flicking lavishly beautiful short dancing skirts back from net-stockinged long legs.

Throughout most of this experience, although there was no actual music, there was symbolic, whirling, interpretive dancing to music felt rather than heard, music beaten out in a mad, crazy primitive tempo. At one time I saw and was part of fish life in shimmering opalescent water but I saw no actual fish. Rather, I felt their presence. A flush of translucent purple red was exuded from some form of marine life and flowed in quivering waves through the rippling water, punctuated with silvery bubbles, which rose slantingly to the surface. I felt the shimmery movement of gliding through the non-resistant quality of the water.

I was briefly exploding volcanoes and with each eruption my body violently shuddered and shook. Then I saw and was great mountains crashing and tumbling into a foaming sea far below. Through a long stillness, I heard the for-

lorn beseechingly lonely sobbing of all childhood, restricted inner sobbing held within by an agony of repression. Then came the deep cries of weeping adults, men and women, and moaning and groaning. I saw a blue face, drawn in anguish with the mouth open and arms outstretched; then a multitude of contorted weeping faces with matted hair and knobby work worn hands out-stretched. And throughout the pitiful wailing of sobbing childhood in an agony of repression and loneliness. Although I cried very little during this experience I was wracked and torn inside with sobbing, exactly as I was through the long years of my own lonely childhood when I was not permitted the relief of tears or the solace of loving arms.

After this passed the volunteer immediately wanted to paint. She chose large sheets of heavily textured Fabriano paper and recklessly poured out huge globs of paint onto the palette. Normally she was much more frugal, as these supplies are expensive. With tremendous energy, abandon, and an exhilarating freedom, she painted using large brushes heavy with paint and water. She felt that she knew exactly where each color should be placed and she painted with tremendous confidence, sureness, and enjoyment.

In the painting I poured out the surging emotions boiling inside of me. Quickly I did two paintings and then felt completely drained, depleted. They were much wilder and freer and more colorful than anything I had ever done before and I liked them enormously. I didn't actually paint the Kachina doll but the paintings occurred, nevertheless while looking at the doll through eyes col-ored by the emotions I was experiencing. I couldn't have done otherwise.

U.R.

It was a pure horror experience. Persistent vibrating noise, like a jackhammer beating away in my brain incessantly for a long time. My equilibrium was very poor. I thought this intense series of feelings would never end and that it had been going on for days, for weeks or months.

Another phase. I felt as if I had been totally destroyed and had been turned completely inside out and I could start anew. I realized that the fore-going period of horror had been a necessary thing to tear away the tremen-dously strong wall I had built around myself and now my mind felt itself a liquid free thing, facile as any whim I might have. A new phase more concerned with thinking about myself—Fantasia-type hallucinations, vivid, with music in the background. Mostly black and white trip—Less physical discomfort than before. I thought of a thousand different things in a fleeting instant—childhood memories—beating up bullies of my childhood. Then, as I recalled these incidents, they seemed to have a definite bearing on the formation of my personality and I even said out loud, "So that's why I'm the kind of bastard I am." Then I had a staggering sensation of knowing how it feels to be God. I don't necessarily think I was God but that I was inside Him and knew how it felt to have the power to give life and take it away. (After fantasizing about inserting a speculum in the vagina in my imagination to a long row of females in pelvic position) I have no words to describe part of this feeling. Just that I understood the universe in its entirety and a great feeling of peace and understanding flooded over me as if my soul was washed clean and I had a good look at it. It seemed to be a sort of stomach-shaped organ, black, with a shining nova around it. Rather scarred and dented when I looked closely, but I had been absolved and I had a new lease on it, so a few dents didn't matter.

I began to think about what a rotten SOB I really had been, how many lives I had ruined, including mine, by always taking the easy or expected way out of things when I often knew what the right thing to do was, even though it's harder. A wave of self-revulsion swept over me and I went into the john and sat down and began to look at myself in the mirror. I felt that this was the first time I had really ever seen myself and no one really ever had seen the real me. I don't know how long I sat there and watched that face change a thousand ways, some good, some evil.

BIBLIOGRAPHY

Abramson, Harold A., ed. *The Use of LSD in Psychotherapy and Alcoholism.* New York: Bobbs-Merrill, 1966.

Albaugh, Bernard J., and Philip O. Anderson. "Peyote in the Treatment of Alcoholism among American Indians." *American Journal of Psychiatry* 131, no. 11 (1974): 1247–1250.

Arieti, Silvano. *Creativity: The Magic Synthesis.* New York: Basic Books, 1976.

Austin, James H. *Zen and the Brain: Toward an Understanding of Meditation and Consciousness.* Cambridge, Mass.: MIT Press, 1998, 2001.

Balandier, G. *Ambiguous Africa: Cultures in Collision.* Paris: Plon, 1957.

Benedict, R. *Patterns of Culture.* London: George Routledge and Sons, 1934.

Bergman, R. L. "Navajo Peyote Use: Its Apparent Safety." *American Journal of Psychiatry* 128 (1971): 695–699.

Brecher, Edward M., and the editors of *Consumer Reports Magazine.* "The Consumers Union Report on Licit and Illicit Drugs." Mount Vernon, N.Y.: Consumers Union, 1972.

Calabrese, Joseph D. "Spiritual Healing and Human Development in the Native American Church: Toward a Cultural Psychiatry of Peyote." *Psychoanalytic Review* 84, no. 2 (1997):237–253.

Caldwell, W. V. *LSD Psychotherapy: An Exploration of Psychedelic and Psycholytic Therapy.* New York: Grove Press, 1969.

Chandler, A. L., and M. A. Hartman. "Lysergic Acid Diethylamide (LSD-25) as a Facilitating Agent in Psychotherapy." *Archives of General Psychiatry* 2 (1960): 286–299.

Cohen, Athur, A. "Redemption." In *Contemporary Jewish Religious Thought,* eds. Arthur A. Cohen and Paul Mendes-Flohr, 761–765. New York: Charles Scribner's Sons, 1987.

Cohen, Sidney. *The Beyond Within*. London: Paladin Books, 1964.

D'Aquili, Eugene, and Andrew B. Newberg. *The Mystical Mind: Probing the Biology of Religious Experience*. Minneapolis: Fortress Press, 2001.

Dean, S. *Psychiatry and Mysticism*. Chicago: Nelson Hall Publishers, 1975.

de Rios, Marlene Dobkin. "The Non-Western Use of Hallucinogenic Agents." In Vol. 50 of *Drug Use in America: Problem in Perspective*. Appendix, 1179–1235. 2nd Report, U.S. National Commission on Marihuana and Drug Abuse. Washington, D.C.: GPO, 1973.

———. "The Influence of Psychotropic Flora and Fauna on Maya Religion." *Current Anthropology* 15, no. 2 (1974): 147–164.

———. "Plant Hallucinogens and the Religion of the Mochica—An Ancient Peruvian People." *Economic Botany* 31, no. 2 (1977): 189–203.

———. *Visionary Vine: Hallucinogenic Healing in the Peruvian Amazon*. Prospect Heights, Ill.: Waveland Press, 1984. Original edition, San Francisco: Chandler Publishing Co., 1984.

———. "Power and Hallucinogenic States of Consciousness among the Moche: An Ancient Peruvian Society. In *Altered States of Consciousness and Mental Health: A Cross-cultural Perspective*, ed. Colleen A. Ward. Newbury Park, Calif.: Sage Publications, 1989.

———. *Hallucinogens: Cross-Cultural Perspectives*. Prospect Heights, Ill.: Waveland Press, 1990. Original edition, Albuquerque, N.M.: University of New Mexico Press, 1984.

———. "Twenty-five Years of Hallucinogenic Studies in Cross-Cultural Perspective. *Anthropology of Consciousness* 4, no. 1 (1993):1-8.

———. "Drug Tourism in the Amazon." *Omni Magazine,* January 1994: 6.

de Rios, Marlene Dobkin, and Fred Katz. "Some Relationships between Music and Hallucinogenic Ritual: The Jungle Gym in Consciousness." *Ethos* 3 (1975): 64–76.

de Rios, Marlene Dobkin, and David E. Smith. "Drug Use and Abuse in Cross-Cultural Perspective. *Human Organization* 36, no. 1 (1975): 15–21.

de Rios, Marlene Dobkin, and Charles S. Grob. "Hallucinogens, Suggestibility and Adolescence in Cross-Cultural Perspective. In *Yearbook for Ethnomedicine and the Study of Consciousness*, vol. 3. Berlin: Verlag fur Wissenschaft und Bildung, 1994.

de Rios, Marlene Dobkin, Charles S. Grob, and John Baker. "Hallucinogens and Redemption." *Journal of Psychoactive Drugs* 34, no.3 (2002): 239–248.

Doblin, Rick. "Pahnke's 'Good Friday Experiment': A Long-term Follow-up and Methodological Critique." *The Journal of Transpersonal Psychology* 23, no. 1 (1991).

Doblin, Rick, and Michael Forcier. "Leary's Concord Prison Experiment: A 34-year Follow-up Study." *Journal of Psychoactive Drugs* 30, no. 4 (1998).

Doblin, Rick, Jerome E. Beck, Kate Obata, and Maureen Alioto. "Dr. Janiger's Pioneering LSD Research: A Forty Year Folllow-up." *Bulletin of the Multidisciplinary Association for Psychedelic Studies* 9, no. 1 (1999): 7–21.

Eliade, Mircea. *Shamanism: Archaic Techniques of Ecstasy.* Translated by W. Trask. New York: Pantheon Books, 1958.

Emboden, William A., and Marlene Dobkin de Rios. "Narcotic Ritual Use of Water Lilies among Ancient Egypt and the Maya." In *Folk Healing and Herbal Medicine.* Eds. G. Meyer and K. Blum. Springfield, Ill.: Charles Thomas Publishers, 1981.

Encyclopedia Judaica. "Redemption." Jerusalem: Keter Publishing House, 1971, 1–9.

Freyre, Gilberto. *New World in the Tropics: The Culture of Modern Brazil.* New York: Alfred A. Knopf, 1959.

Garbarino, M. S. and R. F. Sasso. *Native American Heritage,* 3rd Edition. Prospect Hts., Ill.: Waveland Press, 1994, 483.

Grinspoon, L., and J. B. Bakalar. *Psychedelic Drugs Reconsidered.* New York: The Lindesmith Center, 1997.

Grob, Charles S., and Marlene Dobkin de Rios. "Adolescent Drug Use in Cross-cultural Perspective." *Journal of Drug Issues* 22, no. 1 (1996):121–138.

Grob, Charles S., D. J. McKenna, J. C. Callaway, G. S. Brito, E. S. Neves, G. Oberlaender, O. L. Saide, E. Labigalini, C. Tacla, C. T. Miranda, R. J. Strassman, and K. B. Boone. "Human Psychopharmacology of Hoasca, a Plant Hallucinogen Used in Ritual Context in Brazil." *Journal of Nervous and Mental Disease* 184, no. 2 (1996): 86–94.

Grof, Stanislav. Preface to *LSD Psychotherapy.* Pomona, Calif.: Hunter House, 1994. Original edition, Pomona, Calif.: Hunter House, 1980.

Grof, Stanislav, and Joan Halifax. *The Human Encounter with Death.* New York: E.P. Dutton, 1977.

Halpern, J. H. "The Use of Hallucinogens in the Treatment of Addiction." *Addiction Research.* 4, no. 2 (1996): 177–189.

HarperCollins Encyclopedia of Catholicism. Ed. by Richard P. McBrien. San Francisco: HarperCollins Publishers, 1986, 96–107.

Helman, C. *Culture, Health and Illness.* Oxford: Butterworth-Heineman Publication, 1994.

Hertel, Carl. *Portrait of the Artist with Two Heads. A Study of Stylistic Changes Influenced by the Ingestion of Lysergic Acid Diethylamide.* Catalog. Scripps College Art Galleries, Claremont, Calif., 1971.

Hoffer, Abram. "Treatment of Alcoholism with Psychedelic Therapy. In *Psychedelics: The Uses and Implications of Psychedelic Drugs*. Ed. Bernard Aaronson and Humphry Osmond. New York: Doubleday, 1970.

Hofmann, Albert. *LSD: My Problem Child*. Translated by Jonathan Ott. New York: McGraw-Hill, 1980.

Huxley, Aldous. *Doors of Perception*. New York: HarperCollins, 1990. Original edition, New York: HarperCollins, 1954.

James, William. *The Varieties of Religious Experience*. New York: University Books, 1963.

Janiger, Oscar. "The Use of Hallucinogenic Agents in Psychiatry." *California Clinician* 55 (1959): 251–259.

Janiger, Oscar, and Marlene Dobkin de Rios. "LSD and Creativity." *Journal of Psychoactive Drugs* 21, no.1 (1989):129–134.

Katz, Fred, and Marlene Dobkin de Rios. "Hallucinogenic Music: An Analysis of the Role of Whistling in Peruvian Ayahuasca Healing Sessions." *Journal of American Folklore* 84 (1971): 333, 320–27.

Kleinman, Arthur. *Patients and Healers in the Context of Culture*. Berkeley, Calif.: University of California Press, 1980.

Krippner, Stanley. "Psychedelic Drugs and Creativity." *Journal of Psychoactive Drugs* 17 (1985): 235–245.

LaBarre, Weston. *The Peyote Cult, Fifth Edition*. Norman, Okla.: University of Oklahoma Press, 1989.

Lee, Martin A., and Bruce Shlain. *Acid Dreams*. New York: Grove Press, 1985.

"LSD Pioneers Look Back and Reassess Drug That Shook the World in 1960s," *Los Angeles Times*, 7 March 1979.

Ludwig, Arnold. "Altered States of Consciousness." In *Altered States of Consciousness*. Ed. by Charles Tart. New York: John Wiley & Sons, Inc., 1969.

Masters, Robert, and Jean Houston. *The Varieties of Psychedelic Experience*. New York: Delta, 1966.

McCullough, Michael E., and David B. Larson. "Religious Involvement and Mortality: A Meta-Analytic Review." *Health Psychology* 19, no. 3.

McGlothlin, William H. "Long-lasting Effects of LSD on Certain Attitudes in Normals." Printed for private distribution by the Rand Corporation, May (1962): 16.

McKenna, Dennis J., J. C. Callaway, and Charles S. Grob. "The Scientific Investigation of Ayahuasca: A Review of Past and Current Research. *Heffter Review of Psychedelic Research* 1 (1998): 65–77.

McKinney, Laurence O. *Neurotheology: Virtual Religion in the 21st Century.* Cambridge, Mass.: American Institute for Mindfulness, 1994.

Menninger, K. A. "Discussion: Navajo Peyote Use: Its Apparent Safety." *American Journal of Psychiatry* 128, no. 6 (1971): 55.

Mogar, Robert E., and Robert W. Aldrich. "The Use of Psychedelic Agents with Autistic Schizophrenic Children." *Journal of Psychiatry* 132 (1967): 674–677.

Morley, J., and N. Kay. "Neuropeptides as Modulators of Immune System Functioning." *Psychopharmacology Bulletin* 22 (1986): 1089–92.

Newberg, Andrew, Eugene D'Aquili, and Vince Rause. *Why God Won't Go Away.* New York: Balantine Books, 2001.

Osmond, H. "A Review of the Clinical Effects of Psychotomimetic Agents." *Annals of the N.Y. Academy of Sciences* 66 (1957): 418–434.

Ott, Jonathan. *The Age of Entheogens and the Angels' Dictionary.* Kennwick, Wash.: Natural Products, 1995.

Pahnke, Walter. "The Psychedelic Mystical Experience in the Human Encounter with Death." *Psychedelic Review* 11 (1971).

Pahnke, Walter, and William A. Richards. "Implications of LSD and Experimental Mysticism." *Journal of Religion and Health* 5 (1966): 175–208.

Pascarosa, P., and S. Futterman. "Ethnopsychedelic Therapy for Alcoholics: Observations in the Peyote Ritual of the Native American Church." *Journal of Psychedelic Drugs* 8, no. 3 (1976): 15–221.

Richardson, A., and J. Bowden, eds. "Redemption." *The Westminster Dictionary of Christian Theology.* New York: Atheneum Press, 1983, 487–488.

Schaeffer, Stacey B., and Peter T. Furst, eds. *People of the Peyote: Huichol Indian History, Religion and Survival.* Albuquerque: University of New Mexico Press, 1996.

Schumakere, John F. *The Corruption of Reality.* Amherst, N.Y.: Prometheus Press, 1995.

Seguin, Carlos Alberto. "Folklore Psychiatry." In *The World Biennial of Psychiatry and Psychotherapy,* vol. 1. Ed. Silvano Arieti, 8. New York: Basic Books, 1970.

Siegel, Ronald. *Intoxication: Life in Pursuit of Artificial Paradise.* New York: E. P. Dutton, 1989.

Simon, Herbert A. "A Mechanism for Social Selection and Successful Altruism." *Science* 250 (1990):1665–1668.

Smith, Huston. "Do Drugs Have Religious Import? *The Journal of Philosophy* 61 (1964): 517–50.

———. *Cleansing the Doors of Perception.* New York: Tarcher/Putnam, 2000.

————. "The Good Friday Experiment." In *Hallucinogens: A Reader*. Ed. Charles S. Grob. New York: Tarcher/Putnam Press, 2002.

Stace, Walter. *Mysticism and Philosophy*. London: Macmillan, 1961.

Tart, Charles S. *Altered States of Consciousness: A Book of Readings*. New York: John Wiley & Sons, 1969.

————. *States of Consciousness*. El Cerrito, Calif.: Psychological Processes, 1983.

Tart, Charles, and Allan Smith. "Cosmic Consciousness Experiences and Psychedelic Experiences: A First-person Comparison." *Journal of Consciousness Studies* 5, no. 1 (1998): 97–107.

Taylor-Perry, Rosemarie. "Renewing Ta Hiera, the Holy Mystery Rites of Eleusis." *Shaman's Drum* 60 (2001): 47–60.

Ten Berge, J. "Jekyll and Hyde Revisited: Paradoxes in the Appreciation of Drug Experiences and their Effects on Creativity." *Journal of Psychoactive Drugs* 34, no. 3 (2002): 249–262.

Underhill, Evelyn. *Mysticism: A Study in the Nature and Development of Man's Spiritual Consciousness*. New York: Meridian Books, 1974.

Walsh, Roger, and Frances Vaughan, eds. *Paths beyond Ego*. New York: Tarcher/Putnam, 1993, 94–5.

Wasson, R. Gordon, Stella Kramrisch, Jonathan Ott, and Carl Ruck. *Persephone's Quest: Entheogens and the Origins of Religion*. New Haven, Conn.: Yale University Press, 1986.

Watkins, Harold. "Probing the Mind: Scientists Speed New Drugs That May Help Treat the Mentally Ill." *Los Angeles Times*, 5 March 1979: 1.

Winkelman, Michael. *Shamanism: The Neural Ecology of Consciousness and Healing*. Westport, Conn.: Bergin and Garvey, 2000.

Yensen, Richard, and Donna Dryer. *MAPS Newsletter* 7, no. 2 (1997): 4.

INDEX

clarity as, 8, 9
ego and, 125, 147, 149, 150, 159
first (onset) phase of, 7–8, 9
follow-up questionnaire, 185–92
fourth (recovery) phase of, 7, 9
general population, 215–26
lack of psychotic, 24–25
musician's, 105–7, 126–30, 138–39
negative, 33, 40–42, 43–47, 49–51, 52,
  71–72, 128, 147, 149, 173, 213,
  221–22, 228, 233–34
paranormal phenomena and, 159
positive, 48–49, 53–62, 68–70, 149, 213,
  215–21, 222–33
psychotherapy and, 227–34
Q sort constants for, 32–34, 40–41
religious, 116–18, 165
second (psychological) phase of, 7, 8–9, 12
shift in perceptual frame of reference
  with, 25
spiritual, 8, 9–12, 55–56, 68, 70, 89,
  96–97, 102, 109–10, 116–17, 126–45,
  147, 176, 182, 224, 230–31
subjective, 9–12, 28, 33, 43–63, 215–26
third (diminishing) phase of, 7, 9
twins', 213–14
writer's, 105
Extrovert/introvert, 22, 50

Fang of Gabon, 163
FDA, 4, 74, 174
  halting of LSD experiments by, 2
Fear, 43–44, 103
Flashbacks, 71, 72
40-year follow-up study. See MAPS 40-year
  follow-up study
Freud, Sigmund, 110, 121, 150, 159

Gable, Clark, 24
Garbarino, M.S., 164
Gilbran, Kahlil, 129
God, 131–32, 155, 181, 182, 224
  communication with, 117, 122, 133, 165, 234
  as entheogen, 122, 148
  redemption with, 180–81
  unity with, 119, 122, 134, 135–37, 141,
    145, 230–31
Government policy, 182. See also FDA
Grob, Charles, 161, 162, 174, 180, 182
Grof, Stanislav, 13, 78, 80, 112, 121, 177
Guilt, 45

Hallucinations, 8, 38–39, 41, 43, 47–50,
  90–91, 94–95, 124, 129, 149, 154,

224–28, 232, 234. See also Perception
  neuroscience of, 124, 146
  power of, 156
Hartman, M.A., 146–47
Healing benefits, 164–65
Hertel, Carl, 64–65, 83–87, 108
Hindu (Vedic), 143–44, 148, 155
Hoasca. See Ayahuasca
Hoffer, Abram, 175–76, 177
Hofmann, Albert, 5
Huichol Indians, of Western Mexico, 166–67
Human history. psychedelics in, 154–57
Huxley, Aldous, 15, 111
Hypersuggestibility, 35, 40

Iboga, 163
Id, 110
Identity, 164. See also Self-concept
  loss of, 71–72
Illegal LSD, 2, 13, 24
Illicit LSD, 13, 23
Indigenous people, 120, 149, 150, 153,
  155–56, 158, 160, 162, 164–67
Individualism, 153, 170, 214, 224
Ineffable, sense of, 35, 39, 142
Inhibitions, 22, 50, 95, 139
Initial follow-up study
  experience variation in, 65–67
  participants of, 64, 65
  queries in, 65
Insight, 70, 136, 232
  artistic, 61–62, 81, 93, 111
  therapeutic, 61, 73, 92, 148, 175, 178–80
Inspiration, 77, 108, 112, 118, 179
Interpersonal relations, 59, 90
Intuition, 70, 97
Irritation, 45–46
Islam, 181

James, William, 116, 120, 121, 146
Janiger, Oscar, 154, 174, 183–84
  academic background of, 14, 25
  art/creativity study of, 2, 22–23, 80–83,
    108–12, 154, 179
  artistic inspiration and, 77, 179
  ego, experience and, 125, 149, 150
  experiments of, 1–2, 4, 6, 8, 9
  follow-up questionnaire of, 185–92
  halting of experiments of, 2–3, 23–24
  MAPS 40-year follow-up study and,
    67–68
  method's of, 19
  mind set of participants for study of,
    17–18, 124–26, 147, 169